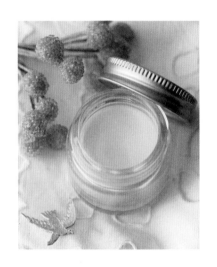

NATURAL
Beauty

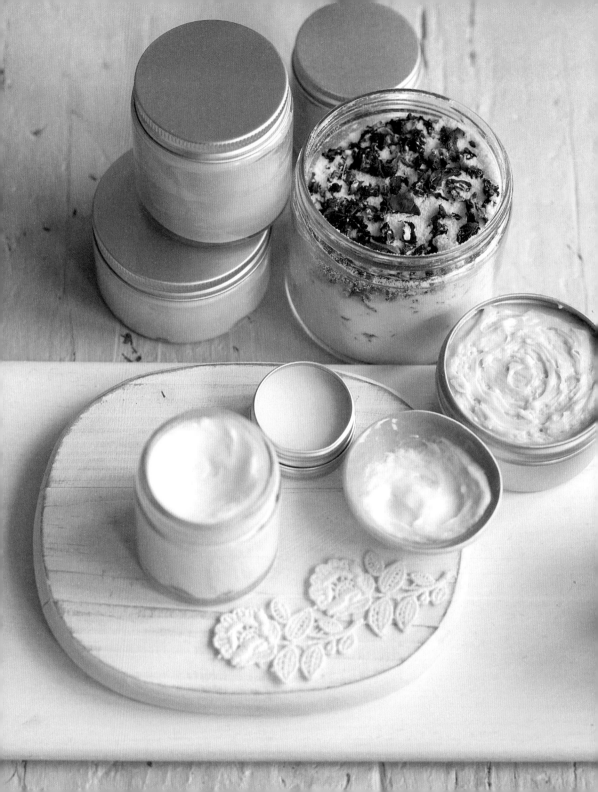

NATURAL *Beauty*

35 STEP-BY-STEP PROJECTS FOR HOMEMADE BEAUTY

KAREN GILBERT

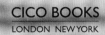

CICO BOOKS

LONDON NEW YORK

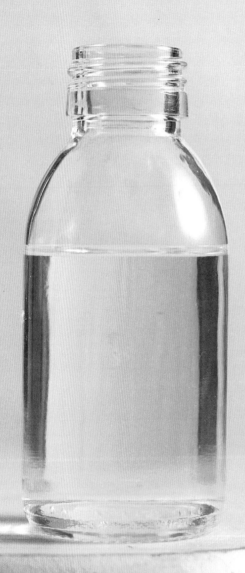

This edition published in 2018 by CICO Books
An imprint of Ryland Peters & Small Ltd
20–21 Jockey's Fields   341 E 116th St
London WC1R 4BW   New York, NY 10029

www.rylandpeters.com

First published in 2011 as *A Green Guide to Natural Beauty*

10 9 8 7 6 5 4 3

Text © Karen Gilbert 2011, 2018
Design and photography © CICO Books 2011, 2018

A CIP catalog record for this book is available from the Library
of Congress and the British Library.

ISBN 978-1-78249-658-8

Printed in China

Copy editor: Alison Bolus
Designer: Louise Leffler
Photographer: Stuart West
Stylist: Sania Pell

Author's acknowledgments
Thanks to the team at CICO Books, Cindy Richards for asking
me to write this book in the first place, and Gillian and Alison
for their tireless editing. Special thanks to Stuart West and
Sania Pell for making the recipes look so beautiful—it was
great working with you both!
    Thanks to my fabulous friends at TCE for all your
encouragement and inspiration, especially Bianca Tait whose
excellent coaching skills helped me to remember how much
I love teaching and sharing my knowledge with others.
    To Romy for believing in me all those years ago, and to
Richie for holding the fort while I took time out to write and for
getting up at the crack of dawn to dig the car out of the snow
so I could get to the photo shoot on time.

Disclaimer
The author and publisher have made every effort to ensure the
accuracy of information in this book and assume no responsibility
for errors, omissions, inaccuracies, or inconsistencies. The safe and
proper use of the recipes and ingredients is the sole responsibility
of the person using them. The author and publisher are not
responsible for any misuse, nor are they responsible for any
allergic reaction. The advice in this book should not be interpreted
as medical advice—any health concerns the user may have should
be addressed by a professional medical practitioner.

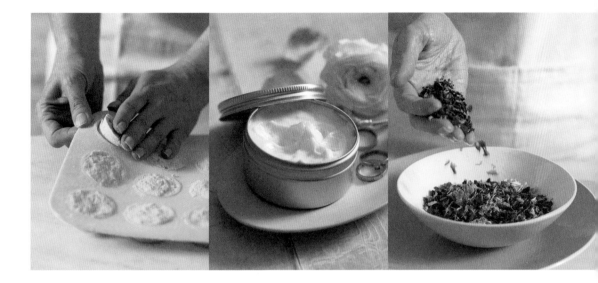

Contents

Foreword by Romy Fraser, founder of Neal's Yard Remedies

In 1981 I founded Neal's Yard Remedies to encourage the use of natural remedies and to support people who wanted to lead healthier, more independent lives.

The company developed a range of toiletries that used the real quantities of traditional beneficial herbs and oils and was constantly seeking alternatives to mass-produced, chemical-based ingredients. My aim was to use natural ingredients to create products that were, and still are, a pleasure to use and that reflected my values of sustainable living. Thirty years later, more and more people seem to share my excitement in making natural skin care products for themselves.

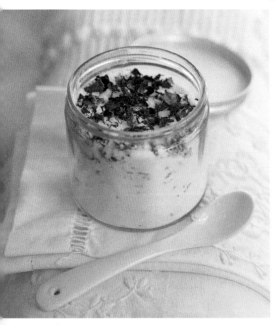

The recipes in this book are a perfect example of ways you can make products yourself without sacrificing any luxuries. I have worked with Karen Gilbert for many years and I am delighted that she has now gathered her wonderful recipes together, to share them with a wider audience. Her recipes are great fun to make, whether you are a complete beginner or simply looking for inspiration.

I am very pleased to recommend Karen's book, and I look forward to using the recipes in our workshops at Trill Farm.

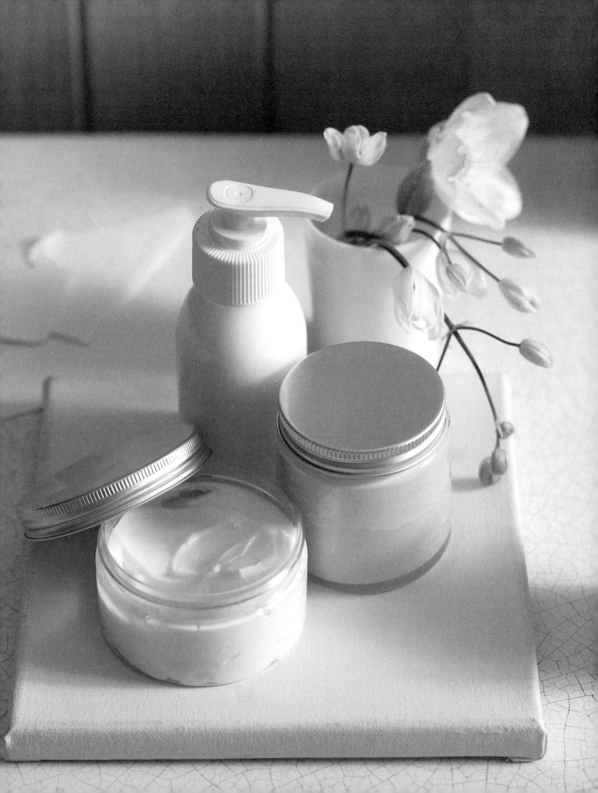

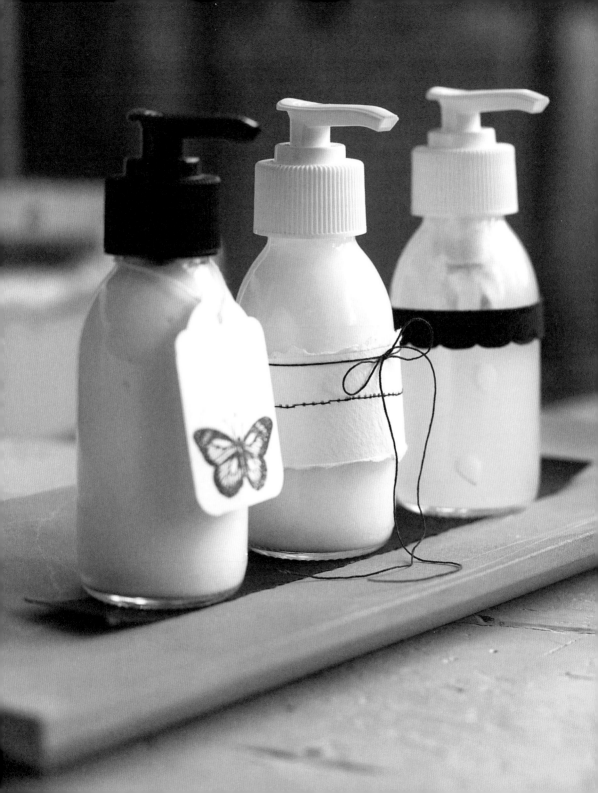

Introduction

After working in the skincare industry for so many years, I sometimes forget that most people do not realize how easy it is to make beauty products at home. There is something I find very therapeutic about hand crafting a product from scratch—just like creating a meal from fresh ingredients, it does take a little bit more time and knowledge than grabbing something off the shelf, but the results are worth it. In writing this book I wanted to create something that could be used both by a complete beginner to make products for fun as well as giving those with a bit of experience some great recipes to try.

The workshops I teach are generally attended by women (and the occasional man) as both a way to learn a new skill and as a social event. Most of the recipes in this book make one bottle or jar of product, but there is no reason why you can't get a group of friends together and make a batch of products. Make it a fun occasion and get creative.

What is natural and is it always best?
My answer is always the same—just because it's natural, it doesn't make it safe and just because it's man made, that doesn't make it harmful. Most ingredients used in skincare are processed in some way to make them usable. Essential oils are steam distilled and oils are pressed by machine. Look for botanical ingredients that have the least amount of processing and are as close to their natural source as possible, and do not be afraid to use a small amount of safe synthetics to make certain products more functional.

The term "green" means different things to each of us depending on our lifestyle. For some it just means recycling and re-using carrier bags; for others it means composting, growing organic veg, and cycling everywhere. When making skincare products, decide on your expectations for their performance and what compromises you are willing to make. For some, emulsifiers and preservatives may be out of the question, which restricts the types of products you can make. For others, you may be prepared to compromise 5–6% of the green-ness for a more sophisticated product—each view is equally valid.

Organic certification has become a huge focus for green skincare brands but I wonder if we have lost sight of some real issues here. Should we be shipping ingredients halfway across the world just because they are organic, and shun good local producers because they do not have organic certification? Should we buy organic over non-certified fair trade, or should we support fair trade co-ops regardless of their organic status? You will need to make up your own mind on what is important to you, and it will be different for everyone.

I hope you find the recipes both fun to make and fabulous to use. Feel free to experiment and if you come up with a great variation, do let me know!

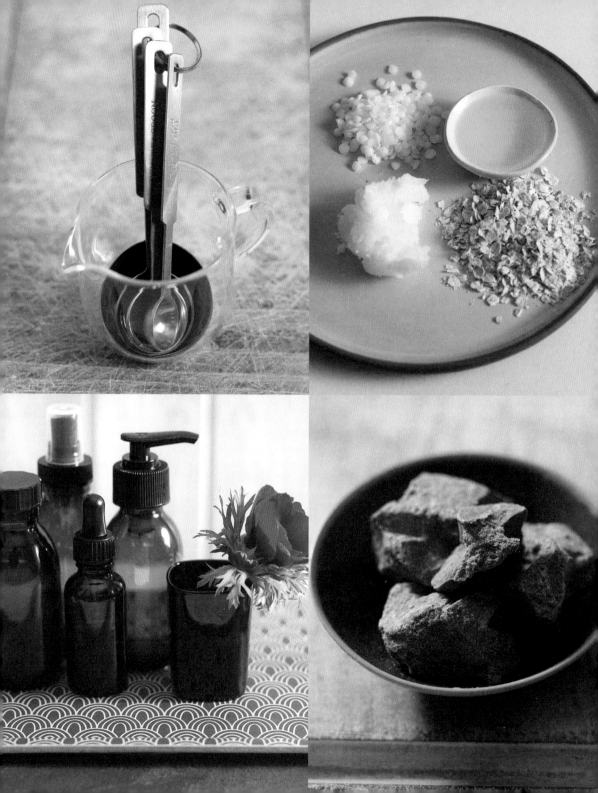

chapter I

Getting started

I know the temptation is to skip this chapter
and move straight on to making the recipes
that follow, but please take just a few moments
to read through these pages. You'll find good
advice on the equipment and different types
of ingredients used in the recipes, plus some
essential information on using preservatives
and the shelf life of your creations. There are
also guidelines on skincare and beauty from
the inside out, and once you've mastered the
basics, you will be able to create your own
variations of my recipes.

Understanding the skin

The dermis

This layer is quite tough with a lot of elasticity since it is mainly composed of connective tissue made up of collagen and elastin. As we age, the collagen fibers—which help to bind water to the skin and give it strength—decline, and so wrinkles start to develop. If the skin is overstretched, as in cases of obesity and pregnancy, the elastin fibers can rupture, resulting in stretch marks. The dermis also contains hair follicles, sweat glands, sebaceous glands, blood and lymph vessels, and sensory nerve endings.

The sebaceous glands are located near the hair follicles and are present in all parts of the body except the palms of the hands and soles of the feet. They secrete sebum—a mixture of oils and fats—in order to keep the skin lubricated and to provide some waterproof protection. Sebum also acts as a bactericidal and antifungicidal agent to prevent microbes invading the skin. Sebaceous activity is regulated by the male sex hormone androgen, which is present in both men and women and increases at the onset of puberty; this is why oilier skin and acne are more common around that age, especially in teenage boys.

The epidermis

The outermost layer of the skin is itself made up of several layers. The basal layer, at the bottom, also known as the stratum germinativum, is where new cells are created. During their 40-day cycle, the cells move gradually from the basal layer through to the stratum corneum at the surface, where they are sloughed off in a process called "desquamation." New cells will then take their place, and the cycle starts again.

The basal layer is also the site of melanocytes, which are responsible for pigmentation in the skin—the production of melanin. Melanin production is actually your body's defence mechanism against the harmful rays of the sun.

SKIN TYPES

NORMAL
If you are lucky enough to have neither particularly dry nor oily skin, then it could be classed as normal and just needs to be kept clean and hydrated with simple cleansing and light lotions. Many skins fall into what is known as the combination category. Combination skin is where the "T zone" of forehead, nose, and chin is slightly oilier than the cheeks. The cheeks are not necessarily dry, but most of us produce more sebum in the center of the face. Don't be afraid to treat each area with different products, if necessary. If you always seem to have a shiny nose, don't use any moisturizer on it since it is obviously producing plenty of oil on its own.

OILY
Although more prone to blocked pores and blemishes than dry skin, oily skins do have the bonus of looking younger for longer. However, they can also be prone to dehydration and sensitivity, so take that into account when choosing your skincare. Avoid any ingredients that are heavily occlusive, since they may cause breakouts, and include plenty of water-based humectants instead. Choose the lighter oils, such as thistle, rice bran, and jojoba, avoiding coconut oil and butters such as cocoa and shea, because they can block the pores.

DRY
Skins with an under-production of sebum need extra help to stay looking smooth and supple. Adding richer oils and butters to your products helps not only to trap water in the skin but also to smooth the rough edges of the cells in the epidermis, to give a smoother appearance. Cleanse gently and use protective moisturizers in the winter as well as in an air-conditioned environment, since this tends to make dehydrated skin worse.

Three-step skincare routine

The three steps to healthy skin are to keep it clean, to protect it from dehydration and the elements, and to address any problems that occur.

1 Keep it clean

As sebum is sticky, it attracts dirt and debris from the environment and needs to be removed with regular cleansing to prevent pores becoming blocked. You cannot stop sebum production or close the pores, and nor should you want to because they both perform vital functions. For some people, using soap or detergent-based cleansers on the face disturbs the acid mantle of the skin and makes it feel dehydrated and uncomfortable. Here the answer is try a cleansing lotion, oil, or balm instead. As I have an oily skin and like to wash my face with water, I use either a cleansing balm or oil removed with a face cloth or cheesecloth (muslin). For years I used foaming face washes (because I was nervous about using anything oily), but always felt that they irritated my skin. I now use the basic cleansing balm with manuka honey (see p.31), and my skin feels much better for it.

Personally, I do not advocate constant exfoliation with facial scrubs, and think the skin does a pretty good job on its own if treated properly. That said, the act of using a face cloth

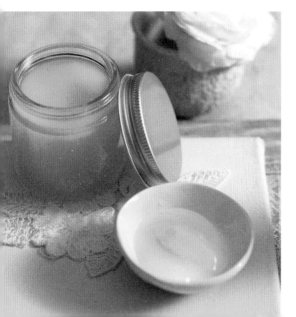

or cheesecloth (muslin) twice a day will remove excess dead cells, so that probably has something to do with it. I would use a scrub only very occasionally if my skin was looking a little dull.

2 Protect it from dehydration and the elements

There are two things you can do to help your skin look and feel better: keep it moist and protect it from trans-epidermal water loss (TEWL). Trans-epidermal water loss simply means that the water in your skin evaporates when subjected to the elements, leaving it dehydrated. Ingredients in skincare products such as humectants have the ability to draw more moisture from the air to the surface of the skin, but they cannot hold it there. This is where ingredients such as emollients and occlusives come in, because they help to slow down the evaporation process whilst keeping the top layer of cells soft and supple. Sometimes we want to create a protective barrier, but if the barrier is too thick it can block the pores and cause spots, so choose your ingredients carefully for your particular skin type.

3 Address any problems

Facial skin problems can be very debilitating. I personally believe that a problem showing on your skin is an indication of something that is out of balance at a deeper level. Conventional medicine and skincare place much of their focus on fixing symptoms and what you can see rather, than investigating the cause. We can all be guilty of this, too, as our primary concern is to get rid of the offending blemish in a quick fix. Whilst this can work in the short term, if the initial cause is not addressed then the blemish, in some form or other, will always reappear.

Addressing skin problems comes back to understanding what is normal for you. For example, I know that my diet, exercise, and stress levels can play havoc with my skin. If they are in balance, my skin is great; if not, then my skin looks dreadful and suffers all kinds of strange pimples. The occasional breakout once a month is normal for me, but anything more than that means I need to get my life back in balance. I visit either a herbalist or a homoeopath for more problematic skin issues, because I do not want to be given antibiotics or steroid cream just to make the problem go away.

Beauty from the inside out

The simplest place to start when aiming for a more green and natural beauty routine is by considering how you look after your body as a whole, as well as the stresses and strains it may be subjected to.

You can have the greatest skincare routine in the world, but it won't make that much difference in the long run if you drink, smoke, and live on a diet of caffeine and junk food while being subjected to constant stress. You would be surprised how many people with skin problems do not even think about changing their lifestyle, and try to fix them with cosmetic products instead.

Diet

What you eat and drink plays a huge part in how you look and feel, and affects everything from your mood to the appearance of your skin.

Try to avoid:

- *Products made with refined white flour and sugar* These are heavily processed, with little nutritional value (and, yes, this category includes white bread, cakes, biscuits, and cookies!)
- *Packaged meals and fast food* These are loaded with sugar, salt, and preservatives, and seem to be the staple diet of many people.
- *A heavily meat-based diet* I am not suggesting that we should all become vegetarians, as that is a personal choice, but try to eat smaller amounts of high-quality, ideally organic, meat rather than large amounts of poor-quality meat.
- *Caffeinated drinks* Caffeine is an addictive drug that messes with your metabolism and dehydrates your body. Kick the habit if you can.
- *Cigarettes* Goes without saying really: premature wrinkles, smelly breath, and a hacking cough are not attractive.
- *Alcohol* It really isn't good for you or your skin, but if you don't want to give it up completely, just make sure it's a very occasional treat rather than a regular occurrence.

Try to:

- *Drink more water* There is much debate about how much water we should drink and how often, but having regular sips of water throughout the day is a great way to keep you hydrated and alert.

- *Make the majority of your diet fresh fruit and vegetables* We in the Western world eat far more refined carbs and protein than is necessary for a healthy diet and not nearly enough fresh fruit and veg. I find that having one or two fresh juices a day along with lots of salads and lightly steamed vegetables ensures I am getting plenty of vitamins and antioxidants in my diet.

- *Incorporate plenty of "good" fats into your diet* Use cold-pressed oils, which are high in essential fatty acids, as well as nuts and seeds.

- *Buy the best you can afford and make as many meals from scratch as possible* We make many excuses for a poor diet based on time and cost, such as "organic food is too expensive" and "I'm too busy to cook every day." It is difficult to juggle work and family and a limited budget with trying to have the healthiest diet, but just do the best you can and take small steps towards changing your eating habits gradually. Buy organic or local produce wherever possible.

Natural remedies

These help to support the body's natural healing ability and aim to work on the root causes of illness rather than just treating the symptoms. The easiest natural remedies to use come in the form of fresh and dried herbs, which you can either buy from a wholefood supplier or grow yourself if you have the space and inclination. Consumed in the form of herbal teas, they also ensure you drink more water as well as gain the added benefits of the herbs. Cleavers, burdock root, and red clover are particularly good for clearing the skin.

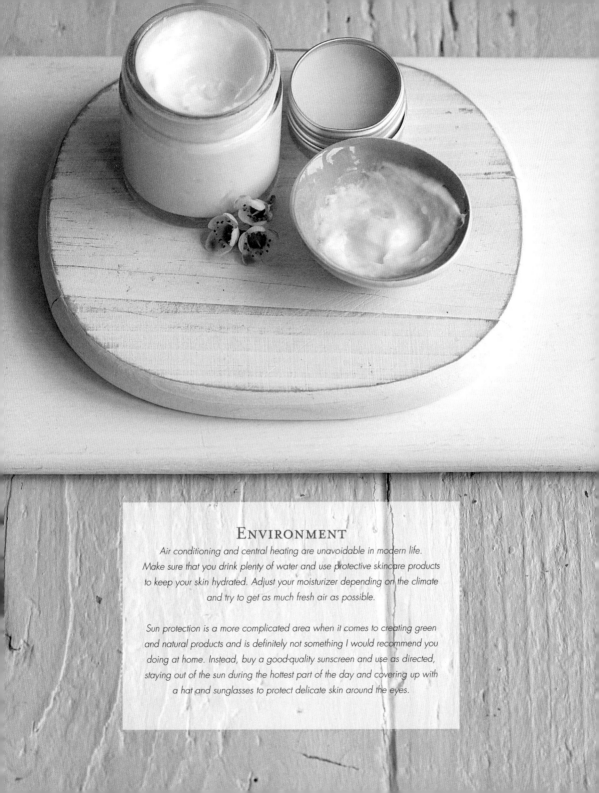

Environment

Air conditioning and central heating are unavoidable in modern life.
Make sure that you drink plenty of water and use protective skincare products
to keep your skin hydrated. Adjust your moisturizer depending on the climate
and try to get as much fresh air as possible.

Sun protection is a more complicated area when it comes to creating green
and natural products and is definitely not something I would recommend you
doing at home. Instead, buy a good-quality sunscreen and use as directed,
staying out of the sun during the hottest part of the day and covering up with
a hat and sunglasses to protect delicate skin around the eyes.

Equipment

None of the recipes in this book requires special equipment that you wouldn't have in your own kitchen, except perhaps a candy (sugar) thermometer. In addition, American readers without a digital kitchen scale will need to acquire one, because weighing ingredients, often in tiny amounts of just 1 gram, is important for accuracy, so cups and spoons will not suffice. Where possible, we have listed many ingredients by volume instead of weight, but not every ingredient lends itself to this treatment. Weighing really is the best option for many of the recipes, and for the soap recipe it is the ONLY option: for safety (getting the lye and water mixture right), all ingredients MUST be weighed accurately.

If you are going to make a lot of products for yourself and friends, I would suggest you buy a set of equipment that you use only for this purpose and never for cooking. The items do not have to be expensive: cheap saucepans, spoons, and bowls are fine. You will also need jars and bottles for your finished products. Rather than reusing food containers, which really isn't very hygienic, you are better off buying new glass jars from one of the suppliers listed on p.143.

You will need:

- digital kitchen scale
- double boiler (one saucepan nesting inside another saucepan, or a heatproof bowl resting over a saucepan; in each case the base saucepan holds simmering water)
- selection of metal mixing spoons and teaspoons (metal is more hygienic and easier to clean than wooden or plastic)
- heatproof glass measuring jug
- milk frother or stick blender (for mixing small and large quantities of creams and lotions)
- measuring spoons
- small glass or metal mixing bowls
- silicone chocolate molds or ice cube trays (for bath melts)
- silicone muffin molds (for massage bars, soap, and bath bombs)
- small plant mister (for bath bombs)
- sifter (sieve) in metal (for bath bombs)
- candy (sugar) thermometer (for lotions and soap)

To make soap, see p.138 for the specific equipment required.

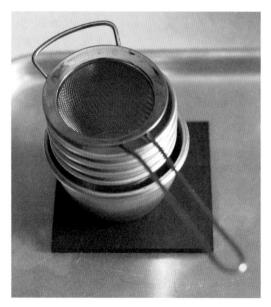

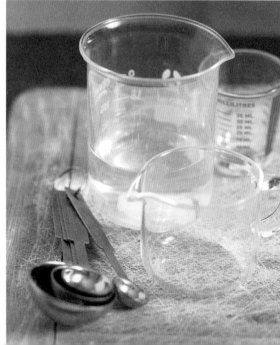

Ingredients

There are many different ingredients that go into natural beauty products, so it is important to know the properties of the ingredients you will be using and why they are necessary. In this section we will briefly cover essential oils and moisturizing ingredients, such as emollients and humectants; as well as the less natural but more functional ingredients such as emulsifiers, detergents/surfactants, preservatives, and antioxidants.

Essential oils

Essential oils are not really oils as such, but highly volatile compounds extracted from fruits, flowers, leaves, roots, woods, and resins, mainly by steam distillation (or expression, in the case of citrus oils). Those materials too delicate to be distilled are usually made into an absolute by either solvent extraction (such as rose absolute and jasmine absolute) or CO_2 extraction. As they are quite volatile and adversely affected by heat, essential oils should always be added at the cooling stage of any recipes that involve heating.

Essential oils are highly concentrated and should never be used undiluted on the skin, as they can cause minor to quite major irritation. There are many oils that are contra-indicated during pregnancy due to their emmenagogue (brings on menstruation) action, though as a general rule I would avoid all essential oils during the first trimester and consult an aromatherapist specializing in pregnancy and birth during later months, when aromatherapy can be extremely helpful.

Dosages

Dosages of essential oils in different product types can vary, but I generally follow the following rules:

- Facial skincare products—a few drops per 3½fl oz (100ml) of product up to a maximum of 0.5%. I have quite sensitive skin on my face, so tend to avoid using more than a couple of drops in a facial moisturizer.
- Rinse-off products, such as shower gels or soaps: 1–2%.
- Leave-on products, such as creams and lotions for the body: 1–2% depending on the oils used and the part of the body. Stick to 1% at first until you know how you will react to a particular oil.   .

Blending essential oils

When blending a fragrance for a product with essential oils, I consider two aspects: What therapeutic benefits, if any, do I want, and what kind of fragrance am I looking for?

Essential oils to start your collection

With this selection you can make a lovely combination of different therapeutic fragrances without spending too much money:

citrus: sweet orange and grapefruit
floral: geranium and ylang ylang
herbal: lavender
resins: frankincense and cedarwood

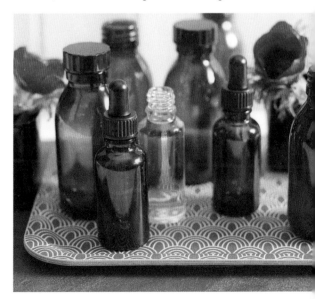

There is absolutely no point in throwing together a bunch of oils that smell terrible when combined just because they are all good for a particular purpose. When I teach natural perfumery, I categorize the oils by both their fragrance family, such as citrus, woody, and floral, and by their volatility, or rate of evaporation—top, middle, and base notes. You will often find that fragrances that fall into the same categories have similar evaporation rates: for example, citrus oils all tend to be top notes and all resins tend to be base notes. To get a balanced fragrance, it is a good idea to include an oil from each of the top, middle, and base note ranges.

I have given suggested essential oil blends for all of the recipes in this book, but do not feel you have to follow them. Fragrance is a very personal thing, so feel free to experiment. You do not need to buy lots of different essential oils, since you can still make great fragrances with just a select few.

Herbal ingredients

Adding herbs to your homemade products is extremely easy. There are several types of herbal extracts that you can buy ready made and some you can easily make yourself. Most commercial skincare products would use a standardized extract rather than adding fresh herbs in the form of an infusion, since infusions do have a tendency to make some products unstable and go off more quickly. If you are making products just for yourself, this shouldn't be a problem, but make sure you do add a preservative when adding herbs to a water-based recipe.

Infusions

Making a water-based extract (or infusion) from the leaves or flowering tops of dried or fresh herbs is as simple as making a cup of herbal tea. Simply add a heaped teaspoon of dried or chopped fresh herbs to a cup or jug and pour on boiling water until it reaches the top. Cover with a saucer and leave to infuse for 10 minutes before straining off the herb matter using a tea strainer or a piece of fine cheesecloth (muslin). Discard the herbs, then add the cooled liquid at the relevant stage in your recipe. If you are making larger quantities of infusions, add one teaspoon of herbs for every cup of water.

Do not keep unpreserved herbal infusions any longer than a day in the refrigerator, as they go off very quickly.

Flower waters

Another way to get water-based herbal extracts into your products is by using flower waters, or hydrolats. These are the byproducts of the steam distillation of essential oils and are very easy to use. Lavender, orange flower, and rosewater are the most common. They make great skin fresheners in their own right and retain the properties of the essential oils from which they are made.

Infused oils

If making an oil-based product, such as a balm or salve, you could macerate your herbs in the base oil used in the recipe. The easiest way to do this is to place a heaped teaspoon of herbs in a bowl and cover them with the base oil of your

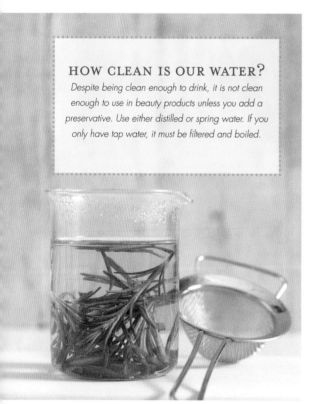

HOW CLEAN IS OUR WATER?

Despite being clean enough to drink, it is not clean enough to use in beauty products unless you add a preservative. Use either distilled or spring water. If you only have tap water, it must be filtered and boiled.

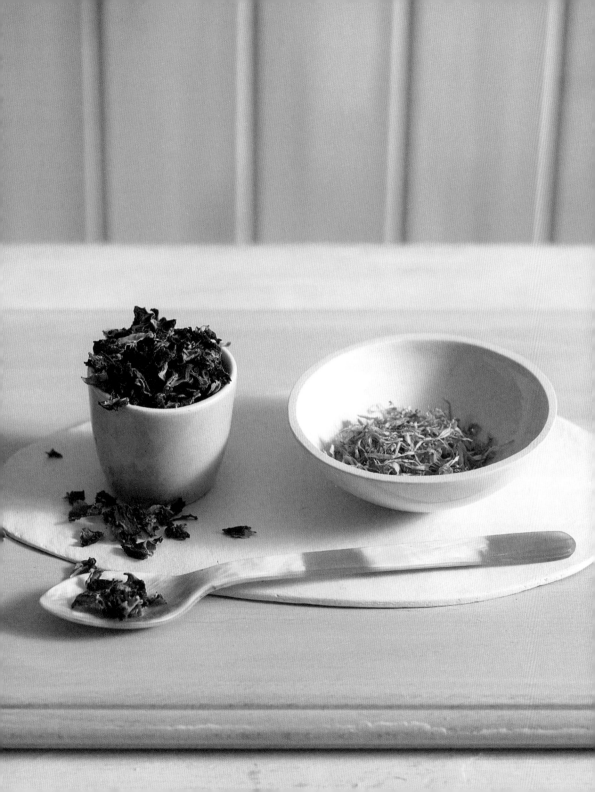

Buying essential oils

Of all the ingredients you will use in your homemade beauty products, essential oils can be the most expensive, so it pays to do your research before spending any money. Rather than spending hours trawling the web for information that is often confusing and contradictory, buy a good book (see my recommendations on p.143) and follow its advice, including the important safety considerations you need to be aware of when dealing with essential oils.

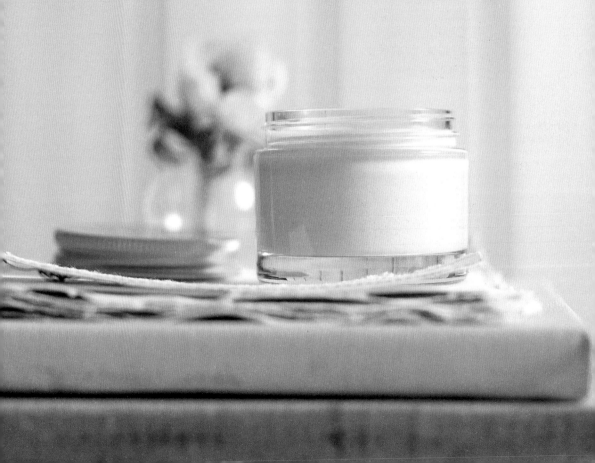

choice. Place this over a saucepan of hot water and simmer for an hour, ensuring the pan does not boil dry. Do not let the oil get too hot: the water, rather than the oil, should be simmering. Strain and discard the plant matter and keep the infused oil for your recipes. Alternatively, buy ready-made infused oils from a herb supplier.

Tinctures, glycerols & CO2 extracts

These final types of extracts are too difficult for most of us to make at home and are best bought from a reliable herbal supplier.

Tinctures are made by macerating herbs for a fairly long period of time in a mixture of alcohol and water. They are primarily sold by herbalists for internal use, but many skincare companies add them to their products. Due to their alcohol content, tinctures may be undesirable for use in products for sensitive skin, as they can have quite a drying effect. The way around this is to use a glycerol (glycerin extract) instead.

The benefit of a glycerol is that the herb is macerated into glycerin, which is both water soluble and a humectant. This means it is suitable for both water-based products and those including an emulsifier, such as creams and lotions. As glycerin is not soluble in oil alone, stick to using oil macerates in products that contain only oils and waxes (or an emulsifier).

CO2 extracts are the result of a fairly new (and expensive) process, known as supercritical CO2 extraction, which is being used to create herb and plant extracts for use in the cosmetic, food, and herbal industries. The plant material is flushed with carbon dioxide under high pressure, which acts as a solvent to release the volatile components of the plant. Due to the lower temperatures involved, it is used as a way of extracting essential oils from plants without the use of chemical solvents when steam distillation is not possible. It is also used to make herbal extracts, which can be added to your products.

Vanilla CO2 extract is particularly useful because vanilla absolute is not soluble in oil and is difficult to incorporate into products, whilst the CO2 extract works perfectly.

Moisturizing ingredients

There are three types of moisturizing ingredients used in creams or lotions—emollients, occlusives, and humectants— and the challenge is to combine them for the best effect. Understanding their basic functions and how they work together will make it a lot simpler to create your own recipes from scratch or to modify any of the recipes in this book.

Emollients

These help to improve the skin's appearance by softening, smoothing, and increasing its flexibility. For my recipes they will be natural plant oils and butters, ranging from the very light and easily absorbed oils, such as thistle, to the richer, heavier butters, such as coconut and shea. Some oils, such as borage and hemp, are rich in essential fatty acids and vitamins but are not particularly emollient and will feel quite dry on their own. For this reason, it is good to include a couple of different oils in each recipe, to improve the performance and skin feel. For each recipe I have included information on the oils so you will have a good idea of what works for different skin types.

Occlusives

These reduce trans-epidermal water loss (TEWL) by creating a waterproof barrier over the skin, and they work best when applied to slightly damp skin. Some emollients, such as cocoa butter, have occlusive properties, along with waxes such as beeswax, which make them great for making barrier products for protecting skin against the elements. Some occlusives are quite comedogenic (acne aggravating) and should be avoided on skin types prone to spots or acne. Many skincare experts are against occlusive ingredients, since it is felt they prevent the skin from breathing; however, for certain areas, such as lips, hands, and feet, they are good for creating a protective barrier on dry cracked skin.

Humectants

Glycerin, honey, and hyaluronic acid are all humectants. Although they are still moisturizers, humectants work in a different way to other moisturizers by attracting water to the skin to keep the cells plump and hydrated. Once the water has been attracted to the skin, you need extra ingredients, such as emollients and occlusives, to keep it there.

Emulsifiers & detergents

Products such as lip balms, body butters, and treatment balms are relatively easy to make, and suitable ingredients can usually be sourced nowadays to make them 100% organic. If, however, you would like to make a more sophisticated cream or lotion, you will need to use both an emulsifier to mix the oil and water-based ingredients together, and a preservative to stop them going off.

Emulsifiers

In simplistic terms, the role of an emulsifier is to make the oil-soluble ingredients stick to the water-soluble ingredients in the same way that you would add egg yolk to oil and vinegar when making mayonnaise. This works because egg yolk contains lecithin, which has emulsifying properties.

If making a lotion or a cream, you would also need to add a thickener to get the texture right, as an emulsifier alone would just create a milky liquid. Some natural emulsifiers that you can buy have thickening properties, but in most cases you would need to add an extra ingredient.

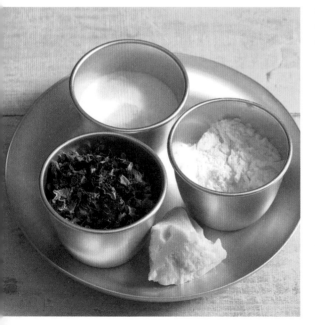

Emulsifying wax

The most commonly found and easy-to-use emulsifier for home use is emulsifying wax, which is a generic term for a number of different formulae. Some types of emulsifying wax contain thickeners and some don't—if you are not sure ask your supplier or simply try out a recipe. If it is too thin and watery you may need to use a separate thickener.

Using emulsifying wax

I have found that using emulsifying wax at 25% of the total fat content without any butters or thickeners creates a thick, but still pourable, lotion. If you want to make a thicker cream, either add slightly more emulsifying wax or add some cetyl alcohol to the recipe.

The alternatives to emulsifying wax

In addition to emulsifying wax, there are many emulsifiers used in the food industry that are available to the home crafter, and you may prefer to use these instead—or at least experiment with them. I have found that for most of the recipes in this book swapping 5% emulsifying wax with 5% glyceryl monostearate plus 2–3% cetyl alcohol works fine, although it does give a slightly thicker texture. I have also included a recipe suitable for oily skin (see p.46) using a new (and possibly the greenest on the market to date) emulsifier—Olivem 1000—that seems to work very well in light lotions.

Ingredient research

If you are at all concerned about an ingredient, do your own independent research because new studies are being done and new information discovered every day. When you read "studies show," try to find the studies and read them yourself.

Detergents/surfactants

If you want to make your own bath and shower gels, you will need to get to grips with a group of ingredients known interchangeably as surfactants/detergents. Most make-at-home recipe books do not cover this type of recipe because these ingredients are seen as evil nasties that should be avoided at all costs. Whilst I agree that the area of detergents and surfactants is a minefield when it comes to being green and eco, I also think it is important to know why ingredients are deemed good or bad. Even if you decide not to make the detergent-based recipes in this book, hopefully you will have a better understanding of the ingredients used and be empowered to make more informed choices when buying over the counter.

There are many naturally derived detergents on the market that are made from sugars, coconut, or palm oil, but please do not be under any illusion that they would just happen to occur without extensive chemical processing. Just because something is naturally derived doesn't make it automatically gentle on the skin and biodegradable, so always check with the supplier you purchase from or look up the INCI names online if you are unsure. (As languages vary around the world, a common language has been devised for labeling requirements, and this means that every ingredient has an INCI name, pronounced "inky"). There is a chance that some ingredients we think of today as "good" and approved by organic certification bodies may, further along the line, come under fire—it is the nature of the industry.

To be as green and eco-friendly as possible, avoid detergents that are:

- *Petrochemical derived* Obviously, as a non-renewable source, anything derived from petroleum should be avoided if you are seeking to be more green.
- *Harsh on the skin* As the whole point of a detergent is to dissolve oil and enable it to be rinsed away with water, many detergents can be quite stripping on the skin and in some cases can be an irritant.
- *Non-biodegradable* If a detergent is not biodegradable, it will stay in the water after being flushed down our drains, damaging both fish and plant life.

So what is a surfactant?

Without getting too technical, a surfactant is a substance that affects the surface tension of water (a surface active agent). It consists of molecules with hydrophilic (water-loving) heads and hydrophobic (water-hating) or lipophillic (oil-loving) tails. In basic terms and in the context of a shower gel, the dirt and oils from the skin stick to the lipophillic end and are lifted away down the drain by the hydrophilic end. Simple!

The detergents I have used in my recipes are the ones commonly used by natural skincare companies that are also readily available to the home crafter. There are plenty more out there, so if you would like more information, look at the resources section at the back of the book (p.143) where I have included the best links I have found for further reading.

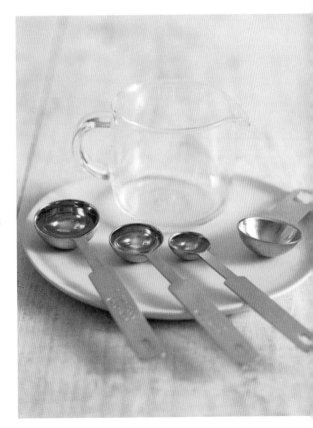

Preservatives & antioxidants

Preservatives

Along with detergents and emulsifiers, preservatives are the cosmetic ingredients that always cause concern for those of us wanting a more green and natural skincare product. To have the phrase "preservative-free" on the label is probably the Holy Grail of natural cosmetics, but it really isn't possible for most commercial products because they are made in huge quantities a long time in advance of sale. This is when making your own cosmetics has definite benefits, as you can make small amounts that need fewer, if any, preservatives.

Any product made using water needs a preservative to stop it going off and becoming both unpleasant and potentially harmful. If you want to avoid preservatives completely, your only choice is to either make products containing no water or to make a very small amount and keep it in the fridge, using within a week or two at the most (see p.26 for more information on making products without preservatives). Products that contain botanical extracts—such as herbal infusions and flower waters—have a much higher risk of contamination by yeast, fungus, and water-borne bacteria, and so need extra preservatives.

Preservatives are placed under constant scrutiny by regulatory bodies, because, by their very nature (killing micro-organisms), they can be harmful to us too. It is quite common to use two or even three preservatives in a blend to ensure that all contaminants are eradicated. For example, some are good yeast inhibitors but are not effective against water-borne bacteria. Other factors that determine the effectiveness of a preservative are the pH of the product and its compatibility with other ingredients, such as emulsifiers and detergents.

Parabens

These are the most controversial of the preservatives. At one time they were used by most skincare companies as they were both effective and unlikely to cause allergic reactions. However, many of the natural skincare brands started reformulating products, due to a study (which has since been discredited) that linked parabens in deodorant to breast cancer. Currently, the American Cancer Society says that there is no scientific evidence that parabens increase the risk of breast cancer, and the FDA considers them safe to be used in cosmetic products. However, just because there is no current evidence, it doesn't mean that there are no long-term effects, and you will need to decide for yourself if you are prepared to take the risk or not. It is worth mentioning that anything that is rinsed off the body, such as shower gel, is less likely to be absorbed into the skin than a leave-on product, such as a cream or lotion.

Suitable preservatives

The other main problems with preservatives are their propensity to cause allergic reactions, plus safety issues such as some being formaldehyde releasers. On p.142 I have listed those available in small quantities for making your own products at home. Although not natural, they are the best available at present. Check out the ones listed and look at the online forums because many crafters are trying different formulations and have interesting experiences to share.

Antioxidants

Many publications quite wrongly call ingredients such as vitamin E and rosemary seed extract "preservatives," when in fact they are antioxidants. So what's the difference?

Oxidation occurs when the product comes into contact with the air and starts to break down or go rancid. Just as an apple turns brown if the skin has been cut, it's a natural process of decay. No outside factors or contaminants need be involved, it's just something that happens naturally as the molecules react with the oxygen in the air. Keeping products in airless packaging and using antioxidants, such as vitamin E and rosemary seed, will slow down this process.

Since products based on oils and waxes are not prone to microbial contamination, they will need only an antioxidant, such as vitamin E, rather than a preservative.

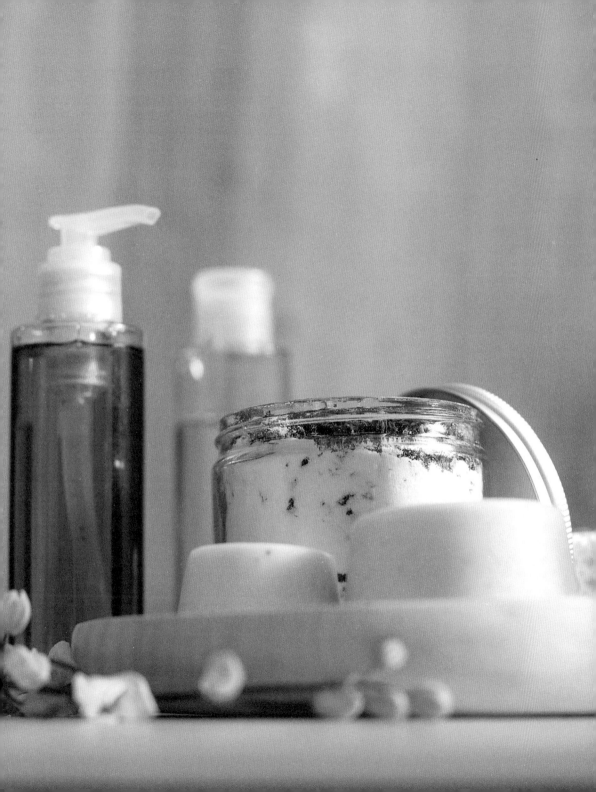

Storage & shelf life
of homemade products

All the recipes in this book include a preservative or antioxidant, where necessary, to prolong the life and freshness of the products—in some cases up to a year or more. I'm sure many of you, however, will want to make fresh natural products using the minimum of chemical additives, so this section gives guidelines on storage and shelf life without preservatives.

A good starting point for prolonging the shelf life of your homemade products is to create a super-clean working environment, using equipment specifically kept for product making that you do not use for cooking. I like to use metal and glass, as they are easy to keep clean and less likely to harbor bacteria. Before you start work, wipe your equipment and countertops with isopropyl alcohol, or rubbing alcohol, which is available from most pharmacies. You could decant a small amount into a spray bottle to mist surfaces and wipe with paper towels; make sure the bottle is clearly labeled and kept in a safe place, as alcohol is flammable.

Creams, gels & lotions

The key thing to remember when working out how long a product will last is whether or not water has been added in any form (this includes bottled spring water and hydrolats, or floral waters). If it has, then the finished product will need to be kept in the refrigerator and will not last for more than a week or two at the most; treat it like a dairy product. The life of a cream or lotion will also depend upon its packaging: if it is in a jar that gets opened every day and has fingers dipped into it, its shelf life will be shorter than a product kept in a bottle with a pump dispenser, which not only keeps fingers out but also prevents air from being sucked back into the bottle. You can buy airless pump dispenser packaging from some ingredients suppliers.

If you are adding herbal ingredients to your products (especially infusions), this will also reduce the shelf life,

since they are a great growing medium for bacteria. If you notice mold growing on the top, thinning or separating of the product, strange smells, or changing color, throw it out!

Lip balms, butters & salves

These are products that have no water added and are simply made from oils, butters, and waxes. Balm-type products do not grow mold and fungus, but they will eventually go rancid over a period of time, depending on the oils used. If you notice a product growing mold, it means that some water has somehow got into it. So, in future, make sure your bottles and jars are completely dry before use.

To gauge how long your product will last, check the expiry dates on the ingredients used and go by the one with the shortest life to be on the safe side. Some oils last a year or two but some, such as rosehip and borage, will turn rancid within a few months if an antioxidant such as vitamin E has not been added at the time of pressing. It is a good idea to buy these oils with an antioxidant already added, if possible. The action of heating the oils and butters during the process of making your products, as well as adding 0.5–1% vitamin E oil (which all the recipes in this book contain), will be enough to lengthen the life of your body butters, salves, and balms to 1–2 years, as long as you are using oils that are within their expiry date.

Face & body oils

These are similar in nature to balms and butters in that they will not go moldy but will oxidize over time and go rancid. As you are not heating them, they will not last quite as long as balms, but they should last a year or so with 0.5–1% vitamin E added (depending on the shelf life of the base oils used). All reputable suppliers should include an expiry date

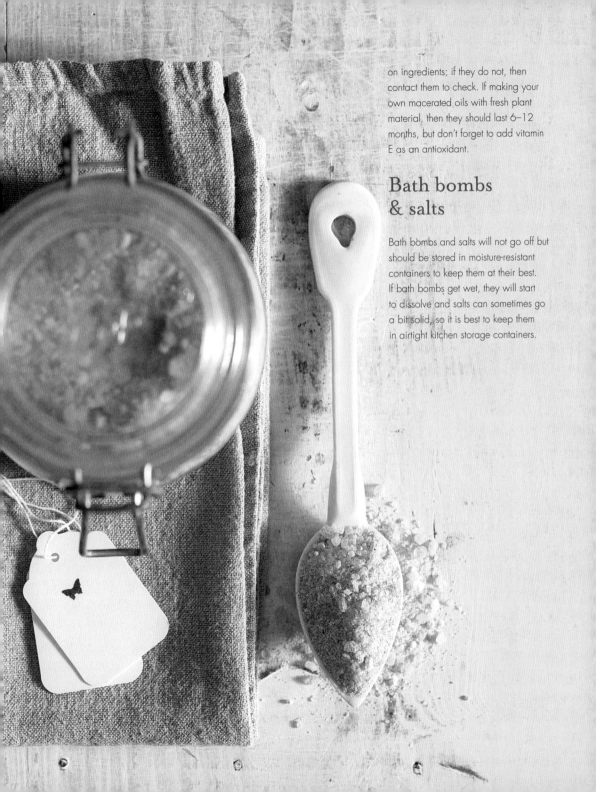

on ingredients; if they do not, then contact them to check. If making your own macerated oils with fresh plant material, then they should last 6–12 months, but don't forget to add vitamin E as an antioxidant.

Bath bombs & salts

Bath bombs and salts will not go off but should be stored in moisture-resistant containers to keep them at their best. If bath bombs get wet, they will start to dissolve and salts can sometimes go a bit solid, so it is best to keep them in airtight kitchen storage containers.

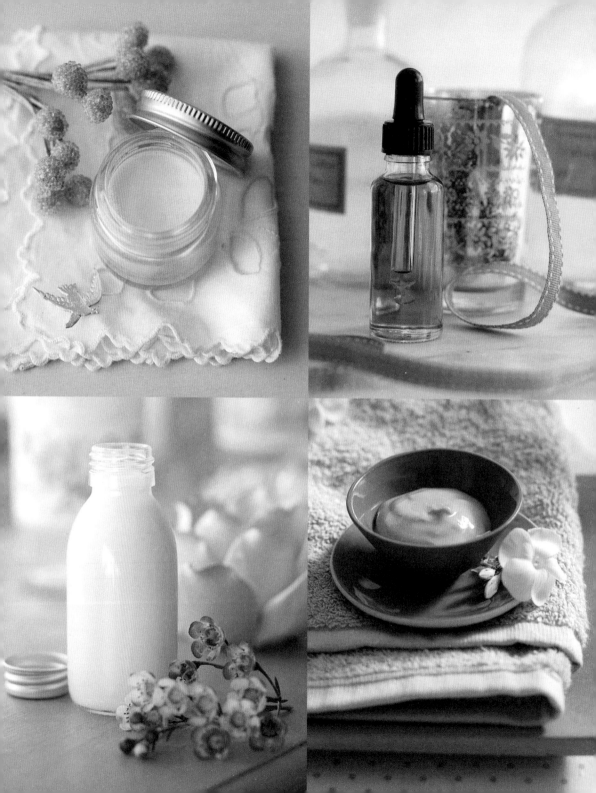

chapter 2

For the face

Skincare products for the face are very simple to
make using good-quality, natural ingredients and can be
just as effective as those bought from a store. Most of us
are much more careful and fussy about the products we use
on our face than we are about those used on the rest
of the body—and quite rightly so, as facial skin is much
thinner and more prone to sensitivity and irritation.
For this reason I tend to avoid using lots of different
essential oils in my facial products and sometimes leave
them unscented or just add a few drops of essential oil
to mask any strong base oil smells. This chapter includes
recipes for everyday cleansers, toners, and moisturizers,
plus special pampering treats, such as face masks, eye
serum, and lip balms.

Rose & red clay cleanser

This fabulously rich and decadent cleanser can be used morning and night to remove make-up and give your skin a pampering treat. It is suitable for dry, sensitive, and aging skin, so if you have an oily or blemished skin, this one may be a bit too rich for you. When blended with patchouli, rose absolute (or, even better, rose otto) is a fabulous anti-aging oil. It is, however, quite expensive, so if you can't stretch to rose, then add a few drops of geranium bourbon essential oil instead.

The role of the jojoba wax here is as a thickener to hold the whole cleanser together. If you do not have jojoba wax, you could just as easily use beeswax, olive wax, or almond wax instead.

Clays make a fabulous additive to cleansers and come in a variety of colors, which all have different minerals and healing properties. The red clay gives the cleanser its gorgeous deep rose color but it is a bit messy to use, so if this is a problem for you, just leave it out or replace it with a different-colored clay depending on your skin type.

Ingredients

10g cocoa butter

20g coconut oil

10g shea butter

10g jojoba wax

4 teaspoons (20ml) calendula oil

2 teaspoons (10ml) manuka honey

10g red clay

3 drops rose absolute

2 drops patchouli

Equipment

double boiler

metal spoon

airtight 3½fl oz (100ml) jar

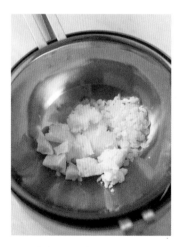

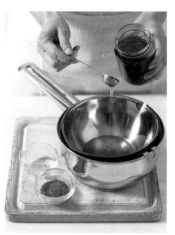

1 Melt the cocoa butter, coconut oil, shea butter, and jojoba wax in the double boiler.

2 Once all the solid ingredients have melted, add the calendula oil and honey and stir gently with the metal spoon until everything is liquid. (The honey will not dissolve fully but will mix into the blend when you add the clay in the next step.)

TO USE
Run a clean face cloth or muslin cloth under hand-hot water and place over your face to open the pores. Take a small amount of the cleanser and massage thoroughly into the skin to loosen any make-up and debris. Remove the cleanser with the cloth. For an extra-deep clean (especially if you are wearing make-up), repeat the process.

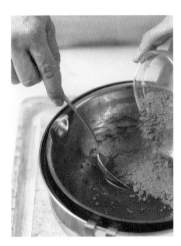

3 Remove from the heat and add the red clay, stirring the mixture gently as it cools to mix in the clay.

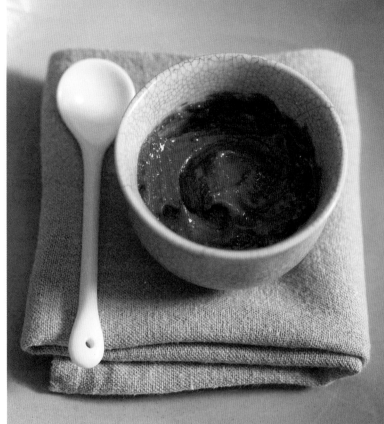

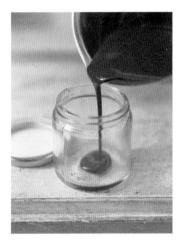

4 Add the rose absolute and patchouli, and stir well. Pour carefully into the jar and seal.

VARIATION

A simplified cleansing balm recipe using your store-cupboard basics:

15g cocoa butter

20g coconut oil

15g shea butter

10g beeswax

2 tablespoons (30ml) almond or jojoba oil

2 teaspoons (10ml) runny or manuka honey

5–10 drops essential oil

Alternatives to rose absolute and patchouli essential oils that you could use are:

Oily skin: lemon, lavender, tea tree

Normal skin: geranium

Dry/Aging skin: neroli, rose

Follow the steps on the left to make this cleanser.

Coconut & oat cleansing lotion

Ingredients

Oil phase

20g coconut oil

2 teaspoons (10ml) castor oil

7g emulsifying wax

Water phase

4 tablespoons (60ml) oat infusion
(see below right)

Cooling phase

20 drops vitamin E oil

20 drops preservative (or according
to the manufacturer's instructions)

10 drops mandarin essential oil

Equipment

cup

tea strainer

double boiler

small glass jug

small saucepan

metal spoon

thermometer

electric (or battery-operated) milk
frother (see equipment chapter)
or stick blender

bowl of cold water

3½fl oz (100ml) bottle with
pump dispenser

Oats are a fabulous ingredient to use on skin, as they produce mucilage when added to water that brings out their soothing and softening properties. Most oat skincare products bought over the counter use a standardized oat extract. Natural or organic skincare companies are likely to use oat (*Avena Sativa*) tincture or CO2 extract, because using an oat infusion would adversely affect the life and stability of the product and warrant a huge amount of preservatives.

Oats are very nutritious for bacteria and fungus as well as to us humans, so make a small amount, keep it in a pump dispenser (so you don't have to keep dipping your fingers in it, which increases the chance of contamination) in the refrigerator, and use it up quickly. Without a preservative, the shelf life of this recipe is minimal (a week in the refrigerator at the very most).

When making a cleanser, it is good to use the more fatty oils as they will not sink into the skin as quickly as some of the drier ones and will be easier to remove. I use food-grade solid coconut oil, which has an amazing aroma, but you could replace it with almond or macadamia oil, which would give a much runnier texture. I have used mandarin essential oil in this recipe as it is very gentle for all skin types and works especially well if you are using coconut oil that retains its natural aroma—it smells good enough to eat!

To make the infusion

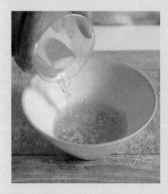 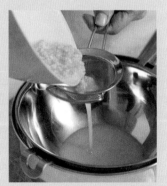

Put 2 teaspoons (10ml) oats in a cup or bowl and pour on 3½fl oz (100ml) boiling water.

Cover and leave to stand for 15 minutes so that the oats infuse the water. Strain through a tea strainer.

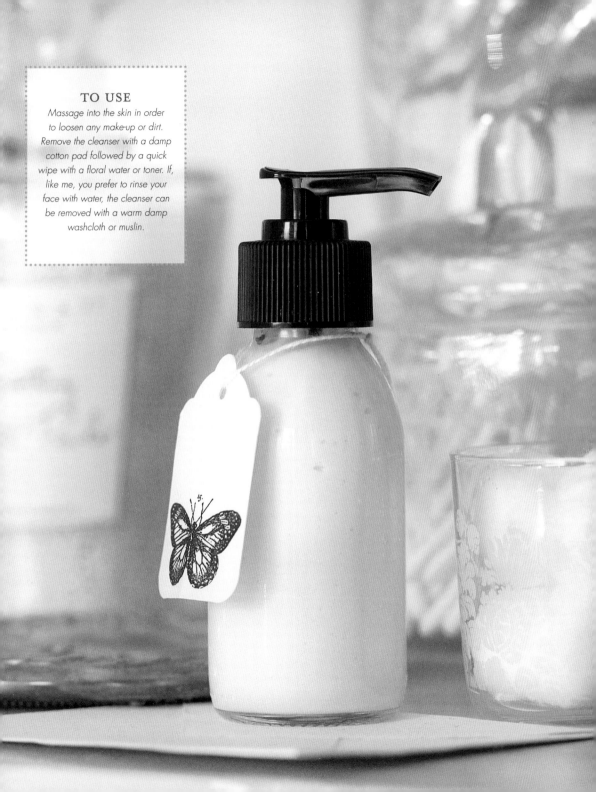

TO USE

Massage into the skin in order to loosen any make-up or dirt. Remove the cleanser with a damp cotton pad followed by a quick wipe with a floral water or toner. If, like me, you prefer to rinse your face with water, the cleanser can be removed with a warm damp washcloth or muslin.

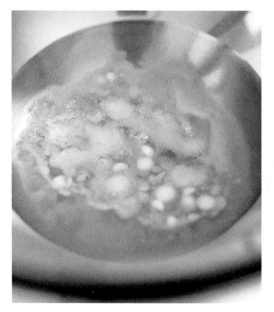

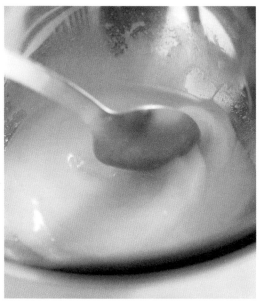

1 For the oil phase, put the coconut and castor oils in the double boiler along with the emulsifying wax.

2 For the water phase, heat the oat infusion in a second double boiler or in a glass jug in a pan of hot water.

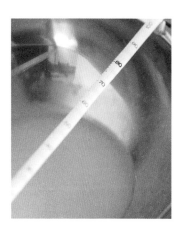

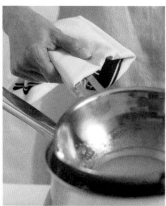

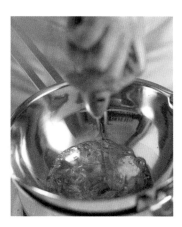

3 Heat until the oil phase ingredients have melted and both the oil and water phase have reached the same temperature of 167–176°F (75–80°C).

4 Remove the water phase from the saucepan of water, taking care not to burn yourself. Always hold with a cloth.

5 Place the milk frother or stick blender into the oil phase, which should still be in the double boiler. Turn on to a low setting, taking care to keep the blender in contact with the base of the pan so as not to introduce too much air into the cream.

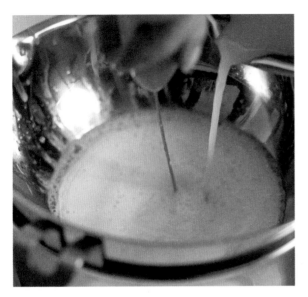

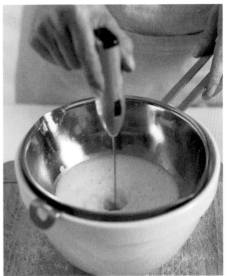

6 In a steady stream, pour the water phase into the oil phase while continually blending with the milk frother. Continue for approximately one minute.

7 Place the jug or pan containing the lotion into the bowl of cold water and continue to blend until the mixture thickens slightly.

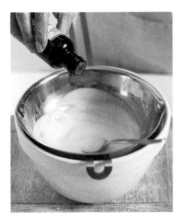

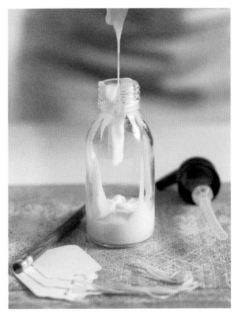

9 Pour into the pump-dispenser bottle. Make sure you label clearly with the date and ingredients used.

8 Once the mixture has cooled, stir in the vitamin E oil, preservative, and essential oil.

Macadamia & jojoba cleansing oil

I'm sure you are wondering why I called this "Macadamia and Jojoba" when the largest ingredient is, in fact, castor oil. Well, the simple fact is that "castor oil" doesn't sound very appealing, and this is an example of why skincare products are often named after their most exotic-sounding ingredient(s) rather than their largest ingredient. However, the manufacturers are not trying to con us, as such, just entice us!

Despite having such an unglamorous name, castor oil is an extremely effective cleanser: it attracts dirt and grime to itself and is very slow to absorb into the skin. It is quite viscous, so it needs to be blended with other oils to allow it to spread more easily; choose other slow-to-absorb oils such macadamia, apricot, or avocado. I have also included jojoba in this cleansing oil, as it is good for all skin types and does not block the pores.

If you intend to use the cleanser to remove eye make-up, then do not add essential oils, because they can irritate your eyes.

Ingredients

2 tablespoons (30ml) macadamia oil

1¼fl oz (40ml) castor oil

5 teaspoons (25ml) jojoba oil

1 teaspoon (5ml) vitamin E oil

10 drops essential oil (optional):

Normal/Dry skin: chamomile, sandalwood, geranium, rose

Oily skin: tea tree, lavender, lemon, cypress, juniper

Equipment

small glass or metal jug

metal spoon

airtight 3½fl oz (100ml) glass bottle with pump dispenser

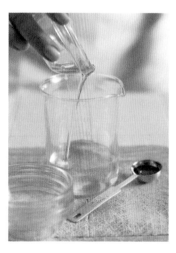

1 Add the oils, one at a time, to the glass jug.

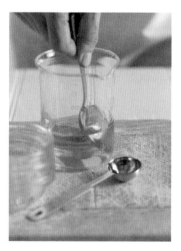

2 Add the essential oils, if using, and mix thoroughly.

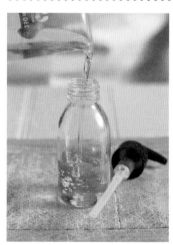

3 Carefully pour into the glass bottle and seal.

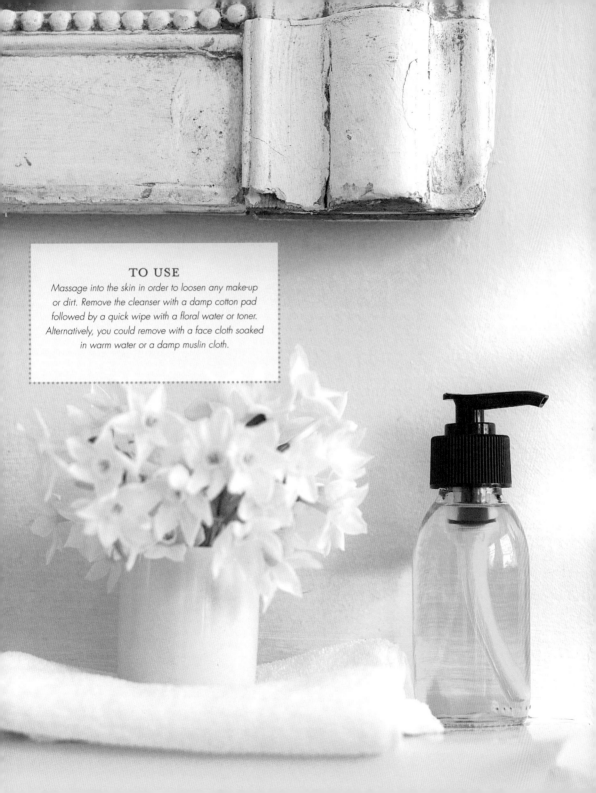

TO USE

Massage into the skin in order to loosen any make-up or dirt. Remove the cleanser with a damp cotton pad followed by a quick wipe with a floral water or toner. Alternatively, you could remove with a face cloth soaked in warm water or a damp muslin cloth.

Lavender & witch hazel skin freshener

Skin fresheners, or toners, are something we were all encouraged to use in the past as part of a cleanse, tone, and moisturize routine, and although they seem to have fallen out of favor, I have included a couple of different options for you here.

If you take a look at the ingredient listing of most good-quality natural toners, they are mainly made up from either water with herbal extracts added or floral waters. Floral waters, or hydrolats, are the byproduct of the steam distillation of plant matter during the production of essential oils. For this reason, it is quite easy to get a huge variety of different flower waters, which can be used as skin fresheners on their own or blended with other water-soluble ingredients. Hydrolats go off quite quickly unless a preservative has been added, so you will usually need to use them within six months.

Witch hazel bark is distilled not for its essential oil but for the sole purpose of producing distilled witch hazel, which has a variety of uses on its own. This hydrolat is great for oily skin, as it is slightly astringent, and it makes an effective eye soother in the summer if you suffer from hay fever.

Ingredients

2 teaspoons (10ml) witch hazel

2¾fl oz (85ml) lavender water

½ tsp (2.5ml) yarrow tincture

½ tsp (2.5ml) vegetable glycerin

Equipment

3½fl oz (100ml) spray bottle

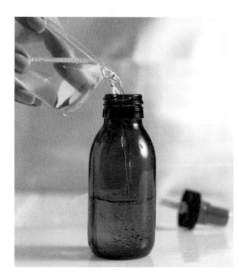

1 Simply measure and pour all four ingredients into the spray bottle.

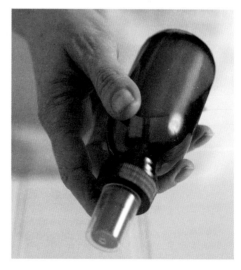

2 Screw the lid on tightly and shake well to mix.

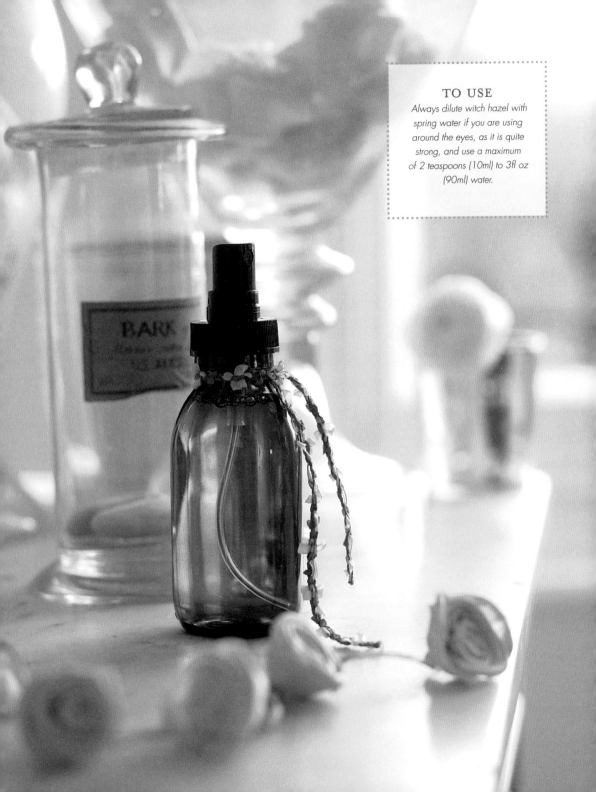

TO USE

Always dilute witch hazel with spring water if you are using around the eyes, as it is quite strong, and use a maximum of 2 teaspoons (10ml) to 3fl oz (90ml) water.

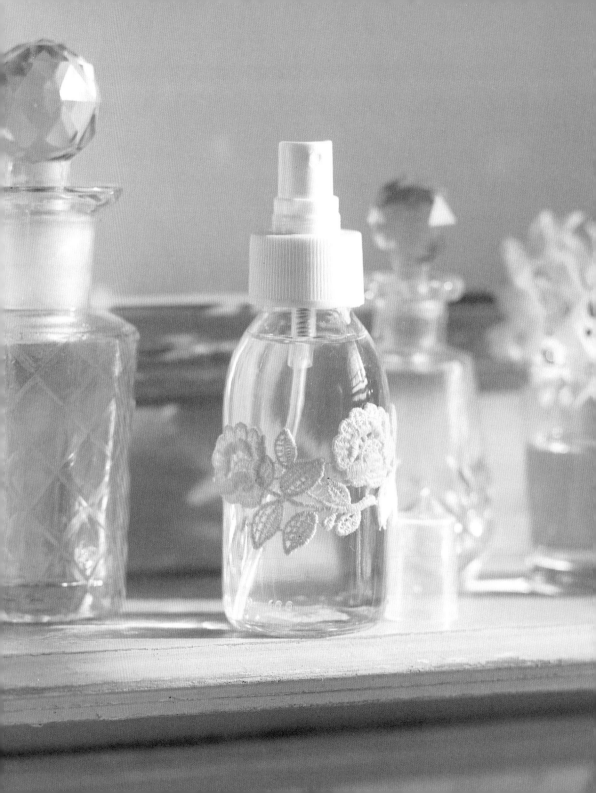

Neroli hydrating spritzer

This hydrating spritzer is along the same lines as a toner, but it is less astringent and more suitable for normal, dry, or sensitive skins. You can add any ingredients to a water-based spritzer like this, but any that are not water soluble, such as essential oils, will float to the top, so you will always need to shake the spritzer before use.

Orange flower water is the byproduct of the distillation of orange blossoms to make neroli essential oil. Both neroli and orange flower water are good for sensitive and aging skin and for those people with broken capillaries.

Aloe vera concentrate is also soothing and can be added to any type of toner or freshener for its anti-inflammatory properties.

I have used vegetable glycerin in this recipe for its humectant properties, but you could replace it with hyaluronic acid, which would be even better.

Hyaluronic acid

Hyaluronic acid is used in commercial anti-aging skincare products and is naturally present in the skin. It can absorb many times its own weight in water and is responsible for giving skin its plumpness and dewy appearance. This naturally diminishes with age, especially after the age of 50, which contributes to the formation of lines and wrinkles.

Note that hyaluronic acid in commercial skincare can be from cocks' combs, but it is also available as a byproduct of bio fermentation, which is the version usually available to the home crafter online (but do check to make sure).

Ingredients

2 teaspoons (10ml) aloe vera

2³⁄₄fl oz (85ml) orange flower water

¹⁄₂ teaspoon (2.5ml) calendula tincture

¹⁄₂ teaspoon (2.5ml) vegetable glycerin

Equipment

3¹⁄₂fl oz (100ml) spray bottle

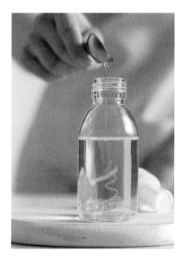

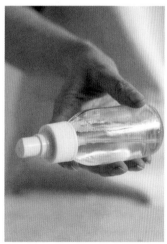

1 Simply add all the ingredients to the spray bottle.

2 Screw the lid on tightly and shake well to mix.

Marshmallow nourishing cream

Like most of the recipes in this book, this one can be adapted for different skin types by adding different oils or herbal infusions once you have mastered the basic process. I have chosen marshmallow (*Althea officinalis*) for this moisturizer for its soothing properties. It is also quite interesting to see how differently it behaves in water to other herbs. The part of the marshmallow plant we will be using is the root, which is available in either a dried or powdered form; when added to water it forms a gel-like substance.

You will notice that in some of the recipes we add an oil in the cooling phase rather than during the heated oil phase. This is because there are some oils whose properties are destroyed by heating, which would make adding the oil at the heated stage pointless. Oils high in GLA and omega fatty acids, such as vitamin E, rosehip seed, and evening primrose, fall into this category, as does borage oil. Keep this in mind if you are replacing any of the oils in the recipes, so that you add them at the correct stage.

Ingredients

Oil phase
2g cetyl alcohol

5g emulsifying wax

2 teaspoons (10ml) macadamia oil

1 teaspoon (5ml) jojoba oil

Water phase
2¼fl oz (70ml) marshmallow infusion

½ teaspoon (2.5ml) glycerin

Cooling phase
20 drops vitamin E oil

20 drops preservative (or according to the manufacturer's instructions)

1 teaspoon (5ml) borage oil

10 drops geranium essential oil

Equipment
small glass jug

tea strainer

double boiler

small saucepan

thermometer

electric (or battery-operated) milk frother (see equipment chapter) or stick blender

bowl of cold water

metal spoon

airtight 3½fl oz (100ml) jar

To make the infusion

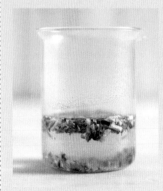 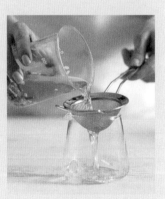

Place 5g marshmallow root in 3½fl oz (100ml) boiling spring water and leave covered for around 30 minutes.

Pour the mixture through a tea strainer and discard the plant matter. Use the infusion in your cream recipe. Any leftover infusion can be stored in the refrigerator for a couple of days.

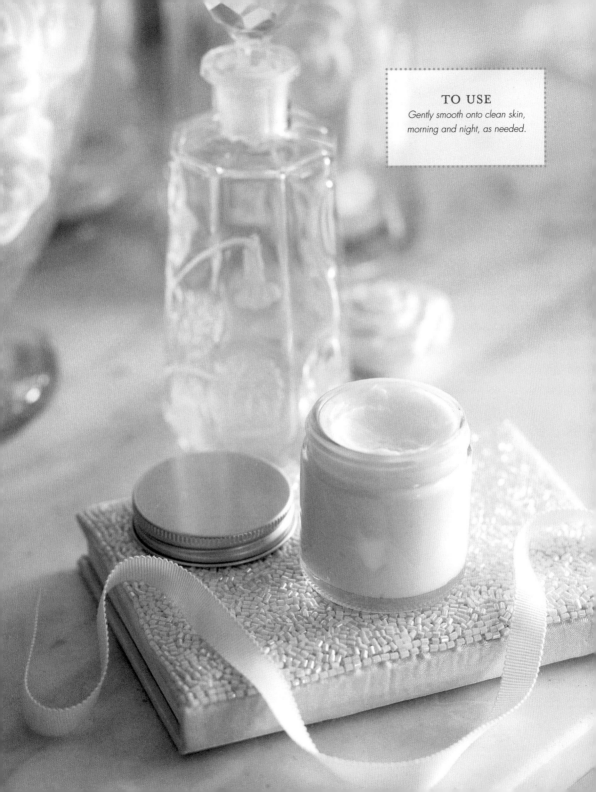

TO USE

*Gently smooth onto clean skin,
morning and night, as needed.*

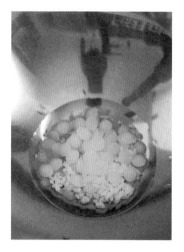

1 For the oil phase, melt the cetyl alcohol and emulsifying wax in the double boiler.

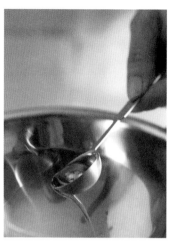

2 Add the macadamia and jojoba oils to the melted emulsifiers.

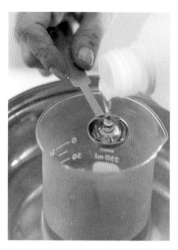

3 For the water phase, heat the marshmallow infusion and the glycerin in a glass jug placed in a saucepan of hot water, or using a second double boiler.

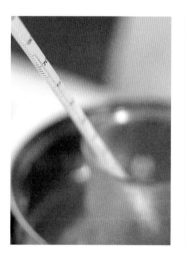

4 Heat until the oil phase ingredients have melted and both the oil and water phase have reached the same temperature of 167–176°F (75–80°C).

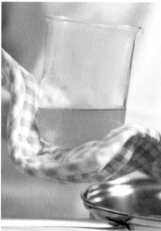

5 Remove the water phase from the saucepan of water, taking care not to burn yourself. Always hold with a cloth.

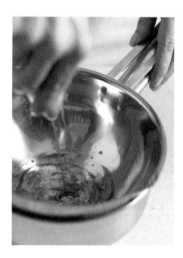

6 Place the milk frother or stick blender into the oil phase, which should still be in the double boiler. Turn on to a low setting, taking care to keep the blender in contact with the base of the pan so as not to introduce any air into the cream.

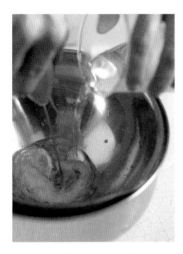

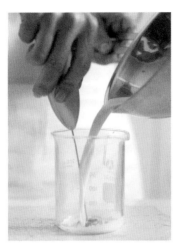

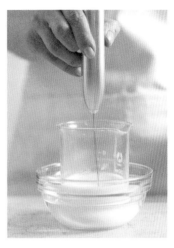

7 In a steady stream, pour the water phase into the oil phase while continually blending with the milk frother. Continue for approximately one minute.

8 You may find it easier at this stage to pour the mixture back into the jug the water phase was in, so it will be easier to pour into the jar later.

9 Place the jug containing the lotion in the bowl of cold water and continue to blend until the mixture thickens slightly.

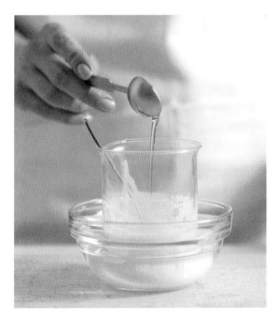

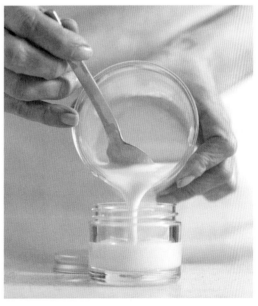

10 Once the mixture has cooled, stir in the borage oil, vitamin E oil, preservative, and essential oil.

11 Pour into the jar. Make sure you label clearly with the date and ingredients used.

Jojoba & aloe vera moisturizer

There are usually two reasons why most of us want to make our own skincare products: either to use fewer chemicals on our bodies or to address a skin problem that commercial skincare or medicine is unable to solve.

As a teenager I suffered from acne due to my oily skin and fluctuating teenage hormones. After trying pretty much everything the doctor or the skincare counter had to offer, at 16 I started dabbling in aromatherapy and making my own face cream. In those days there were very limited resources and ingredients available for making your own products, and most of the recipes included only borax and beeswax as emulsifiers, which made creams too heavy and comedogenic (producing or aggravating acne) for my skin type. It is very important when selecting oils for your creams to use a combination suitable for your individual skin type and an emulsifier to match.

In this recipe I have used a new green emulsifier—Olivem 1000—that is derived from olive oil and at the time of writing is approved for use in EcoCert-certified products. I really like it as you can make very light and almost oil-free lotions from it, since it is water soluble as well as oil soluble.

Ingredients

Oil phase
1 teaspoon (5ml) thistle oil

1 teaspoon (5ml) jojoba oil

3g Olivem 1000

Water phase
2¼fl oz (70ml) spring water

½ teaspoon (2.5ml) glycerin

Cooling phase
2½ teaspoons (12.5ml) aloe vera

20 drops vitamin E oil

20 drops preservative (or according to the manufacturer's instructions)

Equipment
double boiler

small glass jug

small saucepan

thermometer

metal spoon

electric (or battery-operated) milk frother (see equipment chapter) or stick blender

bottle with pump dispenser or airtight 3½fl oz (100ml) jar

Jojoba oil

Jojoba oil is great for oilier skin types, because it is non-comedogenic and helps to balance sebum production. Use it in conjunction with less greasy high-omega vegetable oils such as thistle (safflower) or hemp. Avoid shea butter and cocoa butter, because they are much too heavy for oilier skins and can make spots or acne worse.

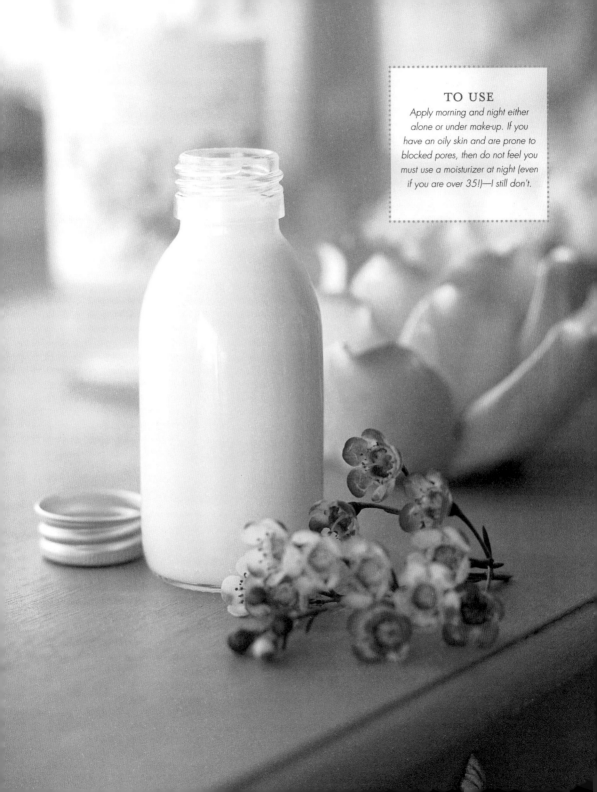

TO USE

Apply morning and night either alone or under make-up. If you have an oily skin and are prone to blocked pores, then do not feel you must use a moisturizer at night (even if you are over 35!)—I still don't.

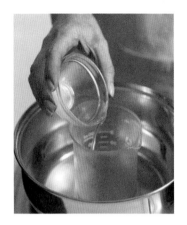

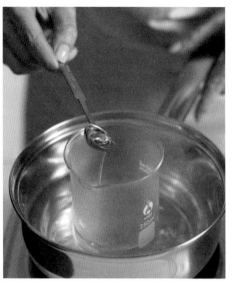

2 For the water phase, heat the spring water and glycerin in a glass jug placed in a saucepan of hot water, or using a second double boiler.

1 For the oil phase, place the thistle and jojoba oil in the double boiler along with the Olivem 1000.

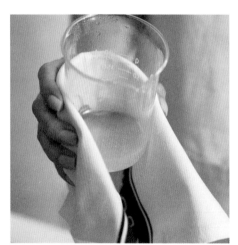

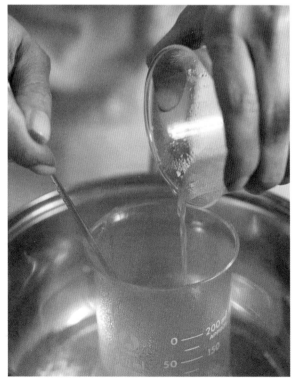

3 Heat until the oil phase ingredients have melted and both the oil and water phase have reached the same temperature of 167–176°F (75–80°C). Remove the oil phase from the saucepan of water, taking care not to burn yourself. Always hold with a cloth.

4 In a steady stream, pour the oil phase into the water phase while continually stirring with a metal spoon. Continue for approximately 2 minutes.

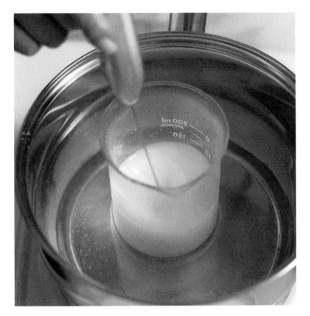

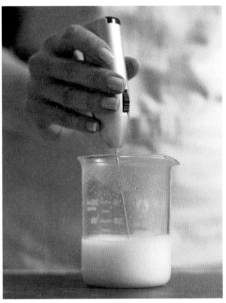

5 Swap the spoon for a milk frother or stick blender and blend for a further 5 minutes.

6 Remove the jug containing the lotion from the heat and continue to blend until the mixture thickens slightly. It is important with this emulsifier to let the mixture cool naturally rather than speeding up the process by sitting it in cold water.

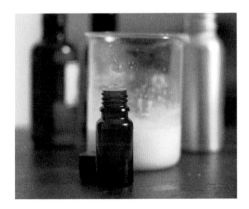

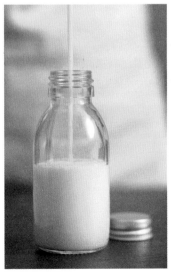

8 Pour into the bottle. Make sure you label clearly with the date and ingredients used.

7 Once the mixture is too thick to blend with the frother, leave it to cool to room temperature. Once the mixture has cooled, stir in the aloe vera, vitamin E oil, and preservative.

Rosehip treatment balm

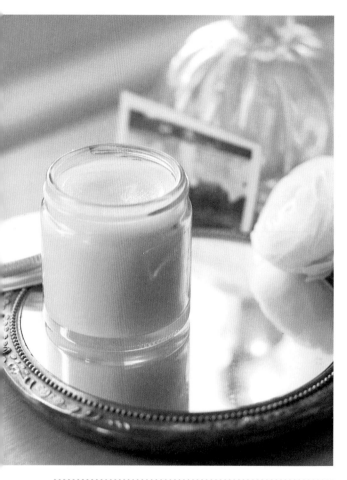

If you want your products to be 100% natural or organic, then the only moisturizer for you is a balm-type product. Balms have no added water, so there is no need for an emulsifier, which means you can add a natural wax such as beeswax or jojoba as a thickener. Beeswax is lovely to use and has a delicious honey aroma, but it does form a heavier barrier on the skin than jojoba wax. I find it a bit too heavy for the face, so stick to using it in hand, foot, and lip products, where the barrier function is needed. If you have a very dry skin and are not prone to spots, then feel free to use beeswax if that's all that is available.

The oils

Rosehip seed oil, sometimes known as rosa mosqueta oil, is usually from Chile. It has excellent skin-regenerating properties and is used for both oily and dry skin types, as well as for helping to heal scar tissue. It is a great oil to use in anti-aging products as well as for skin that has suffered sun damage.

Borage oil is added for its softening properties and high percentage of GLA (gamma linolenic acid), which is thought to help reduce inflammation and accelerate tissue healing to repair and regenerate the skin. It is also sometimes sold as "starflower oil" and is used as a replacement for evening primrose in supplements, since it has a much higher GLA content.

TO USE

This balm is an excellent pick-me-up for tired, stressed skin and can be used on the face or body. Take a small amount on your fingertips and massage gently into freshly cleansed skin. When making the balm, you could pour most into your large jar and then some into a tablespoon-size (15ml) lip balm jar or tin to carry in your purse or handbag.

Ingredients

10g jojoba wax or beeswax

30g shea butter

2 teaspoons (10ml) almond oil

3 teaspoons (15ml) jojoba oil

4 teaspoons (20ml) rosehip seed oil

2 teaspoons (10ml) borage oil

1 teaspoon (5ml) vitamin E

2 drops sandalwood

3 drops rose otto

3 drops geranium

4 drops patchouli

Equipment

double boiler

spoon

airtight 3½fl oz (100ml) jar

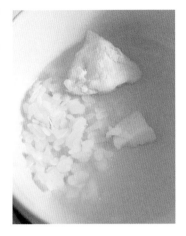

1 Melt the jojoba wax and shea butter in the double boiler. If you have the time, hold the mixture over a gentle heat for about 20 minutes, because this will prevent the shea butter going grainy when it cools. If there is no time, do not worry because it will not affect the performance of the product.

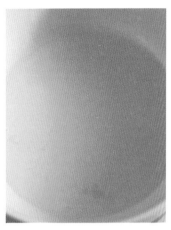

2 Add the almond and jojoba oils and stir gently until everything is liquid.

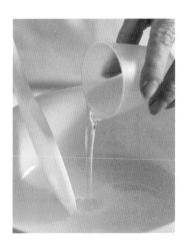

3 As the rosehip seed oil, borage oil, and vitamin E are heat sensitive, remove the mixture from the heat before adding the oils and stirring thoroughly.

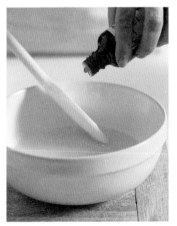

4 Stir in the drops of sandalwood, rose otto, geranium, and patchouli essential oils.

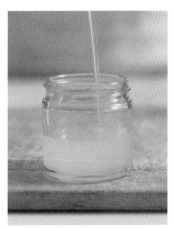

5 Pour carefully into the jar and leave to set.

Regenerating skin serum

The oils used in this blend may be a little unfamiliar to you, but they all are easily available online. If you want to make your own anti-aging skincare products that actually have some effect, then it is worth looking into these speciality oils, which are all jam-packed with vitamins and antioxidants. Look closely at the Latin names and compare them to the ingredients listed on your favorite products: I'm sure you'll be surprised at the similarities.

Note that all of these oils can be incorporated into any lotions you make, too, so don't save them just for the serum.

The oils

Rice bran oil has been used for centuries by Japanese women for its skin-nourishing properties, and it is used to protect against premature aging.

Kiwi seed oil is absorbed into the skin very quickly and doesn't leave an oily residue, which makes it perfect for all skin types.

Argan oil has gained in popularity recently as an anti-aging skin oil. It comes from the argan tree, which grows in certain regions of Morocco. It is very high in vitamin E and linoleic acid.

Pumpkin seed oil has quite a high zinc content as well as vitamins A, C, and E, plus omega-3 and omega-6 essential fatty acids. It is used in skincare and body products for its lifting effect on the skin.

TO USE
Apply a few drops on freshly cleansed skin, either alone or under a moisturizer for an extra boost.

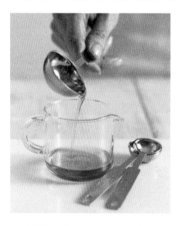

1 Add the oils one at a time to the glass jug.

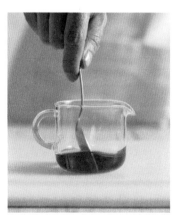

2 Add the essential oil, if using, and mix thoroughly.

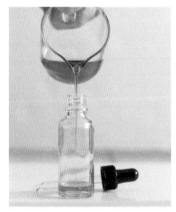

3 Pour the mixture carefully into the glass bottle.

Ingredients

4 teaspoons (20ml) kiwi seed oil

2 teaspoons (10ml) rice bran oil

1 teaspoon (5ml) pumpkin seed oil

1 teaspoon (5ml) argan oil

1 teaspoon (5ml) borage oil

1 teaspoon (5ml) vitamin E oil

5 drops essential oil (optional)

Equipment

small glass jug or beaker

metal spoon

airtight 1½fl oz (50ml) glass bottle
with dropper

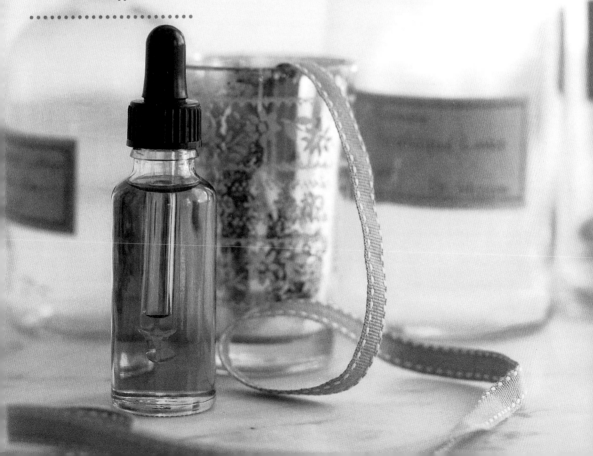

Green clay cleansing mask

When I make face masks for myself at home, it tends to be a spur of the moment thing to use there and then. Clay masks dry out very quickly if you just use water or a herbal infusion, so should really be made in a small quantity fresh for every use. This recipe is for a one-use mask and can be adapted to suit any skin type by changing the essential oils, infusion, and type of clay used—just keep the quantities the same and you will be fine.

This mask is for those times when a cleanser is just not enough. The lavender and juniper oils are both antiseptic and decongesting; the aloe vera will help to soothe inflamed or irritated skin. Green clay is full of minerals and will help to pull the grime and toxins from your pores as well as soothe the skin; it is suitable for all skin types.

Set aside 20 minutes to relax while your mask gets to work on your skin. The best way to do this is to sink into a hot bath, which will also help to open your pores.

Ingredients

2 teaspoons (10ml) lavender water or herbal infusion

½ teaspoon (2.5ml) aloe vera concentrate

1 teaspoon (5ml) green clay

1 drop juniper essential oil

1 drop lavender essential oil

Equipment

small glass bowl or egg cup

spoon

As this is such a small quantity, it is very difficult to weigh the ingredients accurately on most kitchen scales. You will find it much easier to use measuring spoons instead.

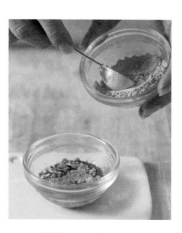

1 Add the lavender water or infusion and the aloe vera to the small bowl.

2 Sprinkle the green clay onto the liquid and stir thoroughly, using the end of a teaspoon.

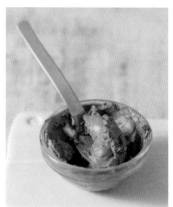

3 If the mixture is still too wet, add more clay; if it's too dry, add more lavender water until you have achieved a nice thick paste that is easy to spread on your skin.

Run a hot bath and wrap your hair in a towel or shower cap. Prepare your mask and apply to freshly cleansed skin, avoiding the eyes and lips; if you have too much for your face, apply the remainder to your neck and chest. Relax in the bath for 15–20 minutes. If the mask starts to feel too tight as it dries, dampen it slightly with water.

To remove the mask, soak a clean face cloth in hand-hot water and place over your face to dampen the mask. Remove the mask with the wet cloth, taking care not to scrub and rinsing the cloth several times.

To finish, either rinse your face one last time with clean water or use the remainder of your infusion or some flower water as a finishing rinse.

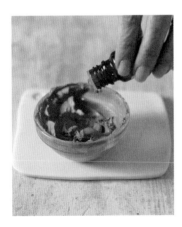

4 Add the essential oils, stirring thoroughly.

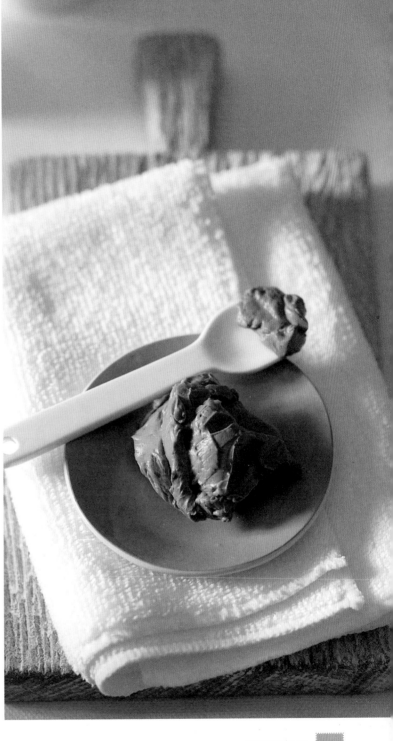

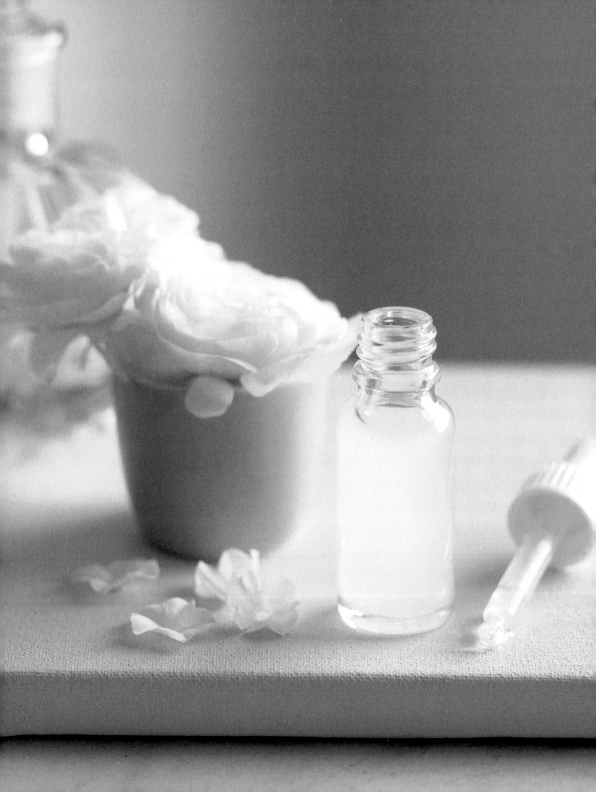

Tea tree spot gel

Tea tree is a great antibacterial and antifungal oil with a multitude of uses, such as in foot products and medicated soap for spotty or oily skin. I do think, however, that its popularity has led to some complacency with its usage and left many people thinking that it is fine just to slap it on neat in great quantities to get rid of spots. In fact it is a very strong oil, and although it can be dabbed onto a spot neat from the end of a cotton bud, I would not advise it—especially on the face, as it can be an irritant to some skins.

As most of us who are prone to spots prefer not to put anything greasy on our face a gel is the perfect medium, and you can vary the thickness of the gel to get the texture that is perfect for you. If you do not want to make a gel, simply add a few drops of tea tree to one of the thin oils, such as thistle or even rosehip seed, which will also help with any scarring.

Ingredients

5 teaspoons (25ml) Basic Gel
(see p.89)

½ teaspoon (2.5ml) witch hazel

½ teaspoon (2.5ml) aloe vera

3 drops tea tree essential oil

Equipment

glass jug

whisk or stick blender

metal spoon

1fl oz (30ml) glass bottle with pump
dispenser or dropper

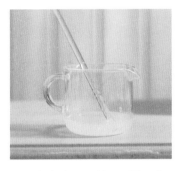

1 Make the basic gel (see p.89) and leave to cool.

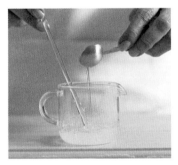

2 Gently stir in the witch hazel and aloe vera.

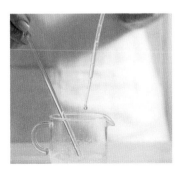

3 Add the tea tree oil and stir gently with a metal spoon.

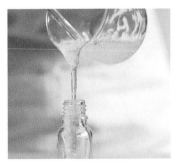

4 Carefully pour the mixture into the bottle.

TO USE
Dab on to the affected area once or twice a day, preferably after cleansing the skin.

Moisturizing vitamin mask

I love using honey in skincare products for its humectant and skin-brightening alpha hydroxy acid properties. Homemade masks (especially those using clay or food ingredients) are best made up in one-use quantities because they do not keep very well. This shouldn't be a problem, since they are quick and easy to whip up just before you need to use them.

This recipe is based on something I originally devised as a training tip for Neal's Yard Remedies' Rose Facial Oil, when I worked for them many years ago. It involved mixing a teaspoon of the oil with some honey and pink clay to make a mask. The oils I have chosen are rich in vitamins (camellia contains A, B, and C, and rosehip seed contains A and C) and antioxidants, and I would recommend using manuka honey.

Feel free to experiment by adding other ingredients to this blend, such as mashed avocado or natural yoghurt if you want a creamier texture.

Ingredients

2 teaspoons (10ml) honey (ideally manuka honey)

1 teaspoon (5ml) aloe vera

1 teaspoon (5ml) camelia oil

1 teaspoon (5ml) rosehip seed oil

½ teaspoon (2.5ml) vitamin E

2–4 teaspoons (10–20g) pink clay or kaolin (white clay)

Equipment

small glass bowl or egg cup

teaspoon

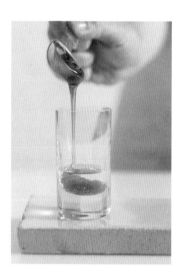

1 Measure the honey and aloe vera into the small bowl or egg cup and mix well.

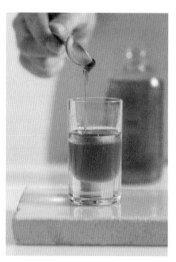

2 Add the camellia oil, rosehip seed oil, and vitamin E, mixing thoroughly with a teaspoon.

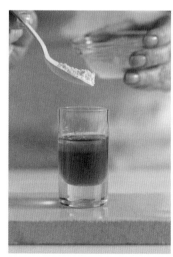

3 Add the clay a little at a time until you reach the desired consistency.

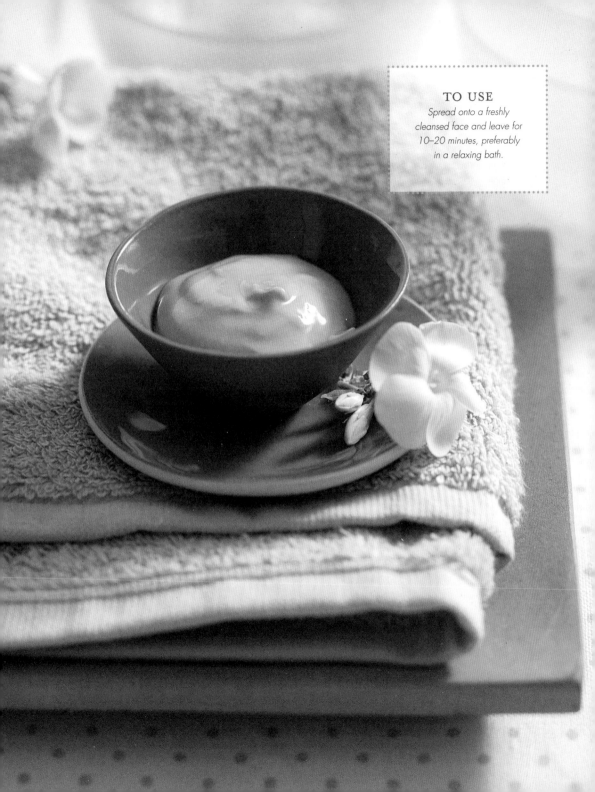

TO USE

Spread onto a freshly
cleansed face and leave for
10–20 minutes, preferably
in a relaxing bath.

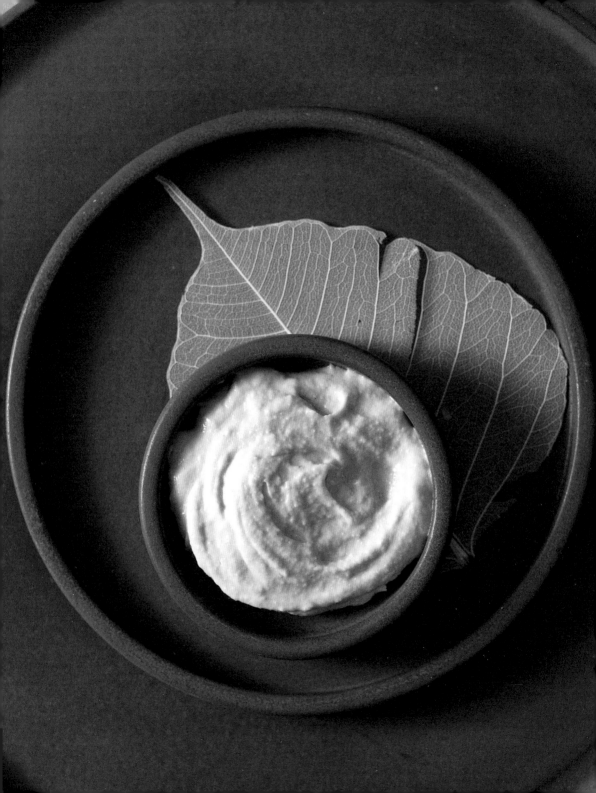

Apricot face scrub

This recipe is one I have used for years to brighten up dull skin. I generally use almond oil because it's what I have mostly to hand, but apricot and castor oils work very well with honey to make a slightly thicker consistency.

   Make up a small amount to use immediately since it does not keep well without preservatives and can separate due to the lack of emulsifier. Using honey and ground rice in a recipe seems to provide a great growing medium for mold, and no matter how careful you are, there is a chance that during usage water from your fingers will find its way into the pot. I make up a tiny quantity and store it in a ½fl oz (15ml) lip balm jar in the refrigerator. This means I use it in a few days and don't need to use a preservative.

Ingredients

1 teaspoon (5ml) apricot kernel oil

1 teaspoon (5ml) castor oil

1 teaspoon (5ml) honey (manuka, if possible)

4 teaspoons (20ml) kaolin (white clay)

½ teaspoon ground rice or rice bran

a few drops orange flower water, if needed

Equipment

small glass bowl or egg cup

teaspoon

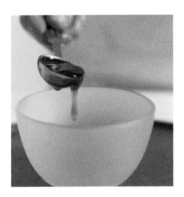

1 Measure the apricot kernel oil, castor oil, and honey into the small bowl or egg cup.

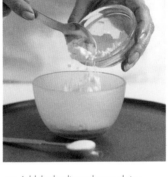

2 Add the kaolin and ground rice or rice bran, mixing everything thoroughly with a teaspoon.

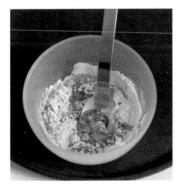

3 If the mixture is too thin or if you prefer a thicker texture, simply add more clay and stir until you get the consistency you want. If the mixture is too thick, add some orange flower water to thin it down slightly. Store any leftover scrub in a small pot in the refrigerator and discard after a few days.

TO USE
Apply a small amount to damp skin and massage in very gently (ground rice can be quite abrasive, so use a light touch). If you find it too harsh or have sensitive skin, try ground almonds instead or jojoba beads, which are available from many online suppliers that specialize in natural product-making ingredients. You can replace the kaolin with green or red clay, if you prefer. To remove the mask, rinse with warm water and a face cloth. This scrub is great to use on the body, too, if you need to use it up.

Argan eye serum

Argan oil is extracted from the kernels inside the fruit of the argan tree, which is found in southern Morocco. It has been relatively unused in skincare until fairly recently, and it can be quite expensive due to the laborious process of extraction and the small yield of the seeds. Traditionally, argan oil was made by the Berber women of Morocco, who gathered the seeds by hand after the fruit had been eaten by goats and the seeds had passed through their digestive system, making them softer and easier to process.

Although oil is still made this way locally, the process has been refined and much of the oil exported is now pressed mechanically by co-operatives set up by the Moroccan government. These programs are dedicated to responsible harvesting and reforestation as well as providing the women of rural Morocco with a fair wage, education, and good working conditions.

If you would like to add a slight lifting or tightening effect to your eye serum, replace an equivalent portion of the vitamin E with ¼ teaspoon (1.25ml) pumpkin seed oil.

Ingredients

1 teaspoon (5ml) argan oil

½ teaspoon (2.5ml) borage oil

1 teaspoon (5ml) rice bran oil

½ teaspoon (2.5ml) vitamin E

Equipment

small glass jug or beaker

spoon or glass stirring rod

½fl oz (15ml) glass bottle with dropper

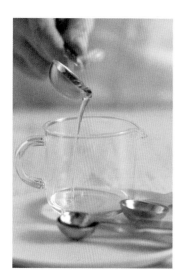

1 Measure the oils one at a time into the glass jug or beaker.

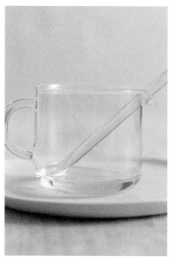

2 Mix the oils together thoroughly, so that they are blended .

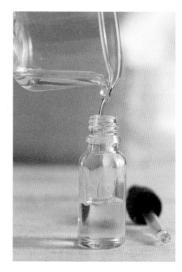

3 Pour the mixture carefully into the glass bottle.

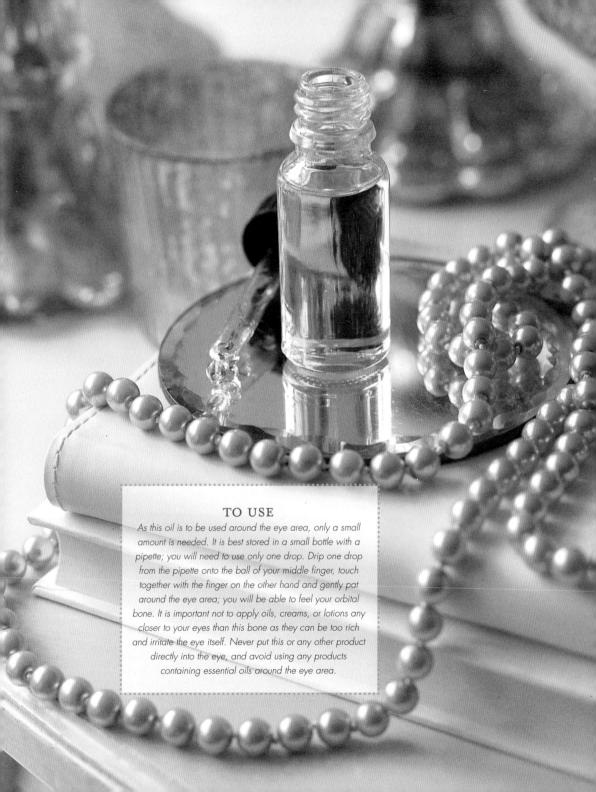

TO USE

As this oil is to be used around the eye area, only a small amount is needed. It is best stored in a small bottle with a pipette; you will need to use only one drop. Drip one drop from the pipette onto the ball of your middle finger, touch together with the finger on the other hand and gently pat around the eye area; you will be able to feel your orbital bone. It is important not to apply oils, creams, or lotions any closer to your eyes than this bone as they can be too rich and irritate the eye itself. Never put this or any other product directly into the eye, and avoid using any products containing essential oils around the eye area.

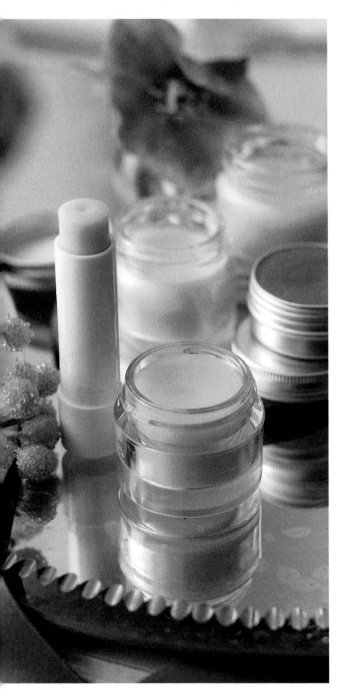

Lip balms

Along with cleansers, lip balms are on the list of products you should never have to buy from a shop again. They come in many guises and it's really easy to make professional-looking products that would also make lovely gifts. With the addition of some fruity natural flavors, they are a good way to engage children in green living. In fact, many of the projects in this book are easy enough to make with children.

The balance of ingredients is a lot more flexible if you are going to put your balms in pots, because you can get away with them being quite soft. You can play around with different oils and butters to find a texture that you really like.

If you want to be more adventurous and use a twist-up stick, then you will need to stick to the oil and wax ratio in the recipe quite strictly because you need a much firmer consistency in order for it to withstand usage in the tube.

Soft butters

You can buy lots of different soft butters online now, ranging from the most common shea butter to mango, apricot, olive, and aloe butter. Of all these, shea butter is the thickest and creamiest and makes, in my opinion, the best lip balm. Cocoa butter is an essential ingredient as it adds firmness but melts instantly on contact with the skin. Beeswax not only holds the whole formula together but also helps it stay on your lips by forming a protective waxy layer.

Hemp & honey lip balm

Honey is possibly one of my favorite skincare ingredients, with manuka honey from New Zealand being the ultimate luxury for its amazing antibacterial properties. Although we are all encouraged these days to buy organic where possible, you do have to look at where the product is produced in order to make the best green choice and take into consideration the distance the product has traveled to get to you.

Due to the very strict guidelines issued by organic certification bodies, it is very difficult for suppliers in some countries to become certified organic producers, which means that most organic honey is imported from producers in Australia and New Zealand. My advice would be to find a local beekeeper from whom to buy honey (and beeswax too, if possible) to help support your local community. If you live in a city you may think it impossible, but beekeeping is more common than you would think—there are many city farms and individual city-based producers with hives. Search for your closest farmers' market where there is bound to be someone selling local honey.

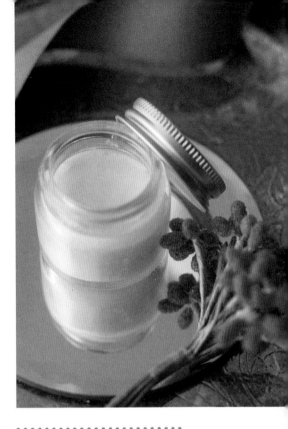

Lip balms

Lip balms are easier to make in batches than individual pots, due to the small quantities used. Most lip balm jars or tins hold around ½fl oz (15ml), although some hold only 1 teaspoon (5ml). This recipe is for four ½fl oz (15ml) jars. If you do just want to make one, then divide the recipe by four.

Ingredients

10g beeswax

10g cocoa butter

15g shea butter

4 teaspoons (20ml) almond oil

1 teaspoon (5ml) hemp oil

2 teaspoons (10ml) honey

Equipment

double boiler

metal spoon

small glass jug

electric (or battery-operated) milk frother (see equipment chapter)

4 x ½fl oz (15ml) jars

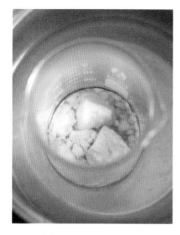

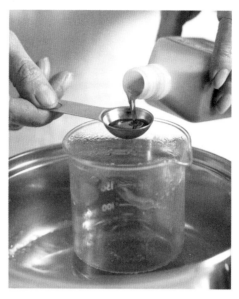

2 Add the hemp oil and honey and stir gently until everything is liquid. As honey is water- (not oil-) soluble, it will not totally dissolve with heating and will need to be mixed in the next step.

1 Melt the beeswax, cocoa butter, and shea butter in the double boiler along with the almond oil.

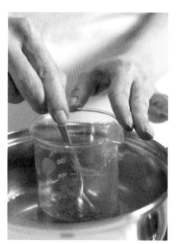

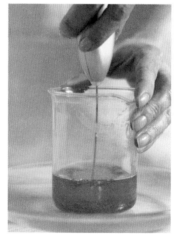

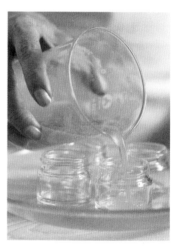

3 Remove from the heat and pour the hot mixture into the jug. Blend with the milk frother for a minute or so until the honey is totally mixed in and the consistency is thicker but still pourable.

4 If you do not have a milk frother, stand the jug in a bowl of cold water and keep stirring the mixture until it cools. As you mix, you will notice the mixture getting thicker and the honey will start to blend in. To help it along, you can put the jug in the refrigerator for a minute or two.

5 Once it is a thick but pourable consistency, pour into the jars to set.

Bee-free lipbalm

For anyone who does not share my love of bee products! Beeswax is replaced with jojoba wax and honey with vegetable glycerin.

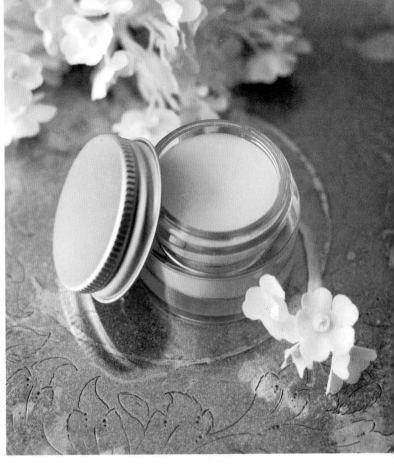

Ingredients

15g jojoba wax

15g cocoa butter

15g shea butter

2 tablespoons (30ml) jojoba oil

4 teaspoons (20ml) hemp oil

1 teaspoon (5ml) vegetable glycerine

Equipment

double boiler

metal spoon

5 x ½fl oz (15ml) jars

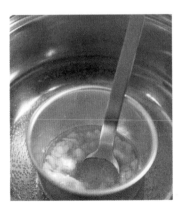

1 Melt the jojoba wax, cocoa butter, and shea butter in a double boiler.

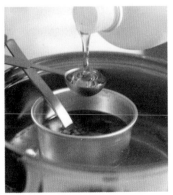

2 Add the jojoba oil, hemp oil, and glycerin and stir gently until everything is liquid.

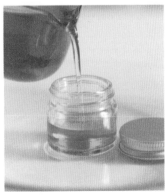

3 Remove from the heat immediately and pour into clean jars to set.

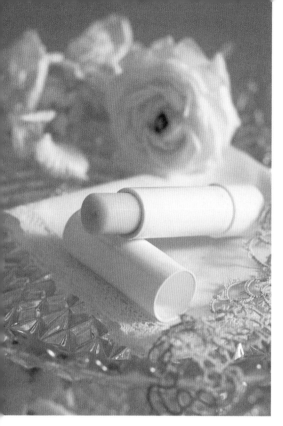

Cocoa butter lip balm sticks

These are a much better alternative to the petroleum-based lip balm sticks available commercially. Lip balm sticks need more beeswax to keep them firm enough to twist up, and they also need a little practice and a steady hand to fill the tubes. Most suppliers listed on p.143 stock the tubes, which are usually either 4.5g or 5g. It's easier to make a batch of five than to weigh ingredients for just one since the amounts are small, but if you do want to just make one simply divide the ingredients by five and melt in a small shot glass or egg cup in a bowl of hot water instead of using a double boiler.

When filling the tubes, it is important to place them in a tray of ice-cold water and to fill them just a quarter full at first to form a plug in the base. If the mixture does not cool fast, it will leak out of the bottom of the tubes. If the mixture sets before you have filled all of the tubes, just stand the jug in a pan of boiling water to re-melt, then carry on pouring.

Ingredients

15g beeswax

10g cocoa butter

5 teaspoons (25ml) jojoba oil

(optional) 10 drops spearmint
essential oil or flavoring of choice

Equipment

double boiler

metal spoon

shallow dish or tray of ice cold water
(chill well before starting the recipe)

5 x 5g twist-up lip balm tubes

small glass jug

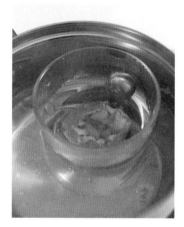

1 Melt the beeswax and cocoa butter in the double boiler.

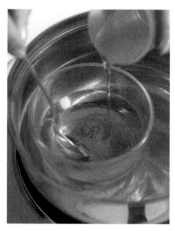

2 Add the jojoba oil and stir until everything is liquid.

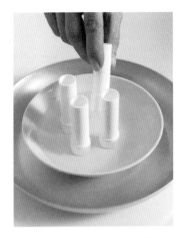

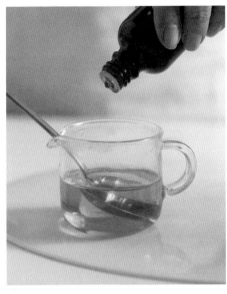

4 Pour the oil and wax mixture into the small glass jug and stir in the essential oil or flavoring.

3 Remove the tray of cold water from the refrigerator and carefully stand the lip balm tubes with the lids off in the water.

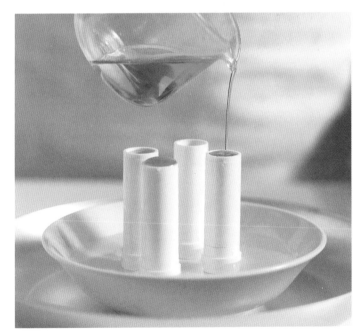

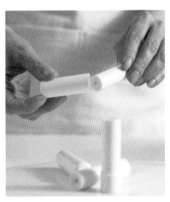

6 Leave to set for 10 minutes or so before putting the lids on, then place in the refrigerator to harden thoroughly.

TO USE
Apply to lips as needed straight from the stick.

5 Let the mixture cool slightly (but not too much or it will set in the jug) before pouring a small amount into each tube (about quarter full). Leave to cool slightly, then top up.

Chocolate orange lip pots

I love using dark organic cocoa butter for lip balm, as it retains its gorgeous chocolate aroma. This recipe contains vegetable glycerin rather than honey, but you could just as easily swap it if you prefer. The flavoring is a lip balm flavor that you can buy online. You could use a food flavor, but you may need to adjust the quantities to taste and check that it is oil soluble. The main recipe is for jars or tins and the variation is slightly more solid for twist-up tubes.

Ingredients

10g beeswax

10g dark cocoa butter

15g shea butter

2 tablespoons plus 1 teaspoon (35ml)
almond oil

1 teaspoon (5ml) glycerin

5 drops orange essential oil

10 drops chocolate flavoring

Equipment
double boiler

metal spoon

small glass jug

5 x ½fl oz (15ml) jars

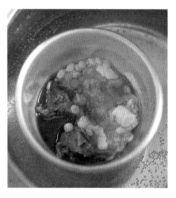

1 Melt the beeswax, cocoa butter, and shea butter in the double boiler.

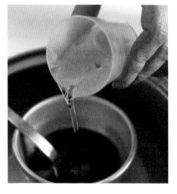

2 Add the almond oil and glycerin and stir gently until everything is liquid.

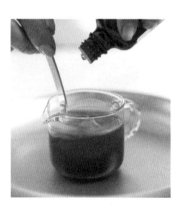

3 Remove from the heat and pour the hot mixture into the jug. Add the orange oil and chocolate flavoring, stirring until slightly cool but still pourable.

4 Carefully pour the mixture into the jars to set.

VARIATION

Follow the method for the Cocoa Butter Lip Balm recipe on p. 68 (makes approx 5 x 5g tubes)

15g beeswax

10g cocoa butter

10g almond oil

15g jojoba oil

3 drops chocolate flavoring

2 drops orange essential oil

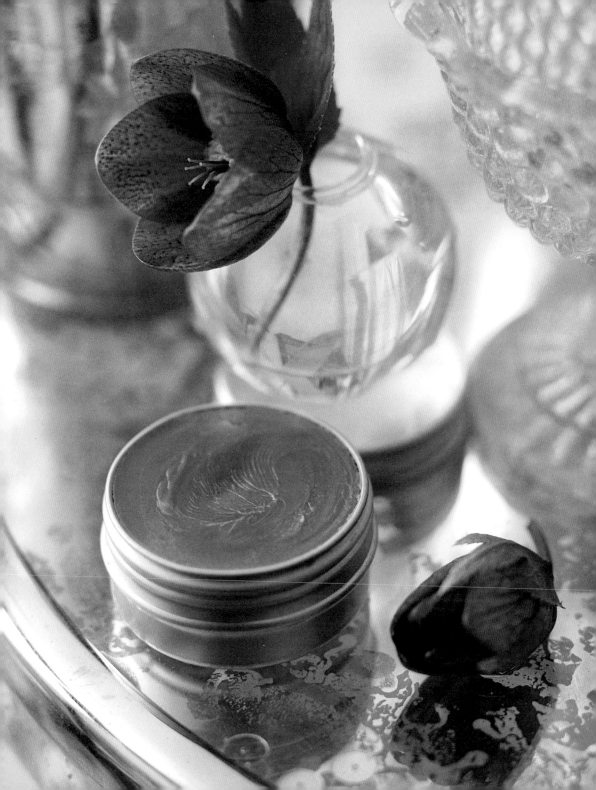

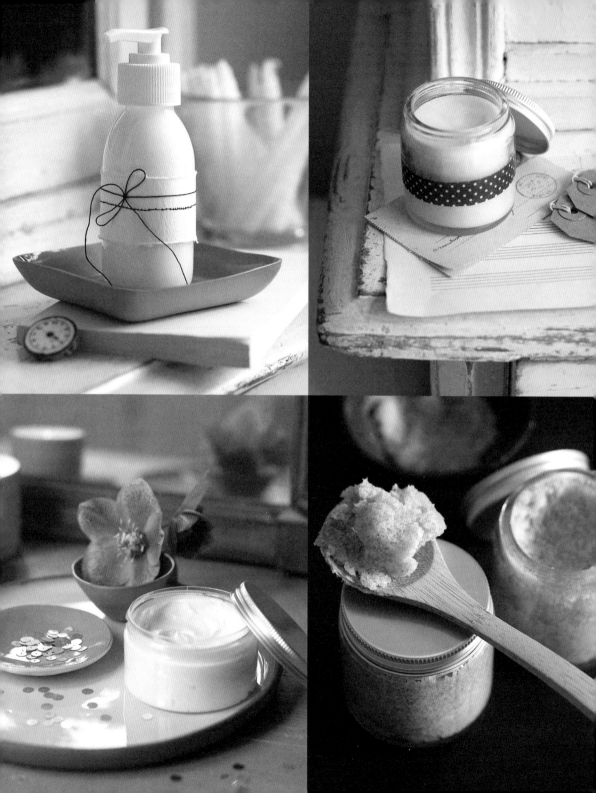

chapter 3

For the body

Body products are, for me, the most fun to make
because you can really go to town with blending your own
fragrances and matching them with your bath products
to create your own personalized range. You can easily
make simple balms and salves from 100 percent natural
or organic ingredients or, with the addition of an
emulsifier and preservative, you can make beautifully
fluffy creams and light lotions for every skin type.
Handmade body products make great gifts too, and
can be decorated with stylish tags and ribbons
for a personalized touch.

Frankincense & orange body lotion

Mmm, frankincense, you could write a whole book on this ingredient alone! From Ancient Egypt to modern times, frankincense (also known as olibanum) has been used both for purifying and clearing the air as well as for its anti-aging and healing properties.

Frankincense essential oil is made by distilling the resin of the *Boswellia* (*thurifera*, *carterii*, or *sacra*) tree, which grows in India, Southern Arabia, and Somalia. The resin is collected by cutting the tree's bark: the sap oozes out of the incisions and forms a solid mass of resin over the tree's wound. Frankincense was used extensively in religious rituals by the Babylonians, Persians, Assyrians, Hebrews, Greeks, and Romans. It was also used by the Ancient Egyptians in rituals, the embalming ceremony, and for making the incense Kyphi. As the olibanum was so precious and considered to be a gift from the gods, it was reserved for placing on the head of the person to be buried.

In modern skincare it is used extensively in anti-aging creams for its ability to help regenerate skin cells, and the boswellic acid found in frankincense is a major component of Boswellox™ used in anti-aging moisturizers.

Frankincense

The scent of frankincense works really well with sweet orange essential oil, which has a joyful, uplifting aroma. Sweet orange is comforting and always makes me feel happy, which I personally believe is an extremely important consideration when choosing essential oils for your own products.

As well as being therapeutic, essential oil blends should be pleasing to the user, otherwise the full benefit will not be gained (my personal opinion by the way, not necessarily a scientifically proven fact!).

Ingredients

Oil phase

5g emulsifying wax

3 teaspoons (15ml) almond oil

1 teaspoon (5ml) apricot kernel oil

Water phase

2¼fl oz (70ml) water or orange flower water

1 teaspoon (5ml) glycerin

Cooling phase

20 drops preservative (or according to manufacturer's instructions)

20 drops essential oils

Equipment

double boiler

small glass jug

small saucepan

thermometer

electric (or battery-operated) milk frother (see equipment chapter) or stick blender

bowl of cold water

3½fl oz (100ml) bottle with pump dispenser

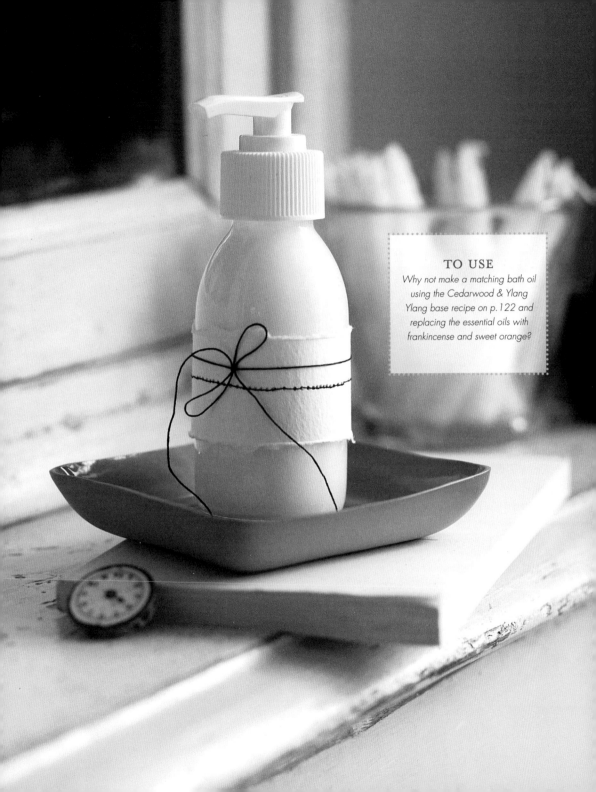

TO USE

Why not make a matching bath oil using the Cedarwood & Ylang Ylang base recipe on p.122 and replacing the essential oils with frankincense and sweet orange?

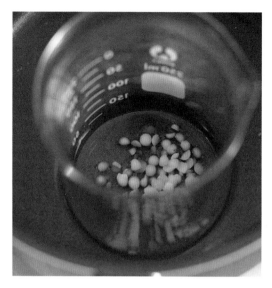

1 For the oil phase, melt the emulsifying wax in the double boiler.

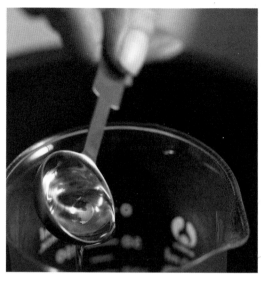

2 Add the almond and apricot kernel oils and heat gently until all is liquid.

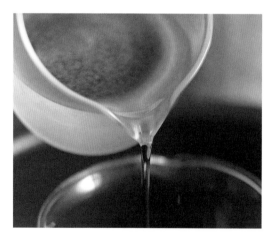

3 For the water phase, heat the orange flower water and glycerin in a glass jug placed in a saucepan of hot water, or using a second double boiler.

4 Heat until the oil phase ingredients have melted and both the oil and water phase have reached the same temperature of 167–176°F (75–80°C).

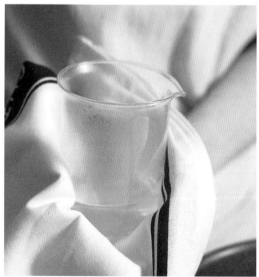

5 Remove the water phase from the saucepan of water, taking care not to burn yourself. Always hold with a cloth.

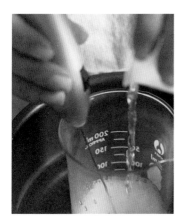

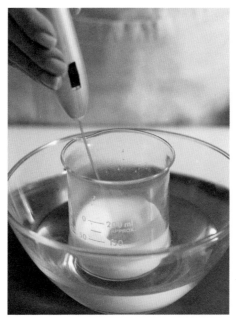

8 Place the jug containing the lotion into the bowl of cold water and continue to blend until the mixture thickens slightly.

6 Place the milk frother or stick blender into the oil phase, which should still be in the double boiler. Turn on to a low setting, taking care to keep the blender in contact with the base of the pan so as not to introduce any air into the cream.

7 In a steady stream, pour the water phase into the oil phase while continually blending with the milk frother. Continue for approximately one minute.

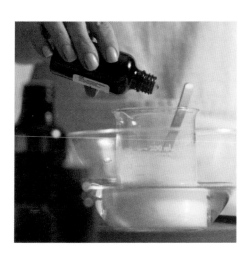

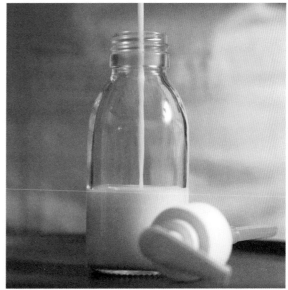

9 Once the mixture has cooled, stir in the preservative and essential oils.

10 Pour into the pump-dispenser bottle. Make sure you label clearly with the date and ingredients used.

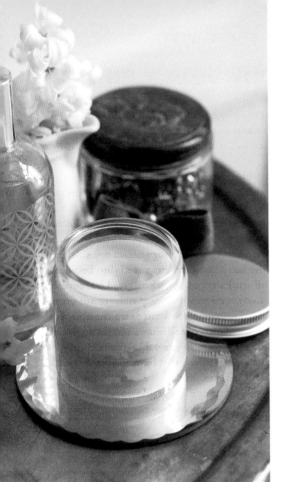

Mango & lime body butter

Mango and lime sounds good enough to eat, although this body butter would work well with any other soft butter, including macadamia, apricot, olive, avocado, or almond. Mango butter is pressed from the kernel of the mango fruit and is used in skincare products for its emollient and moisturizing properties.

The other two butters used in this recipe are more solid, and replacing these will alter the texture of the balm. Both cocoa butter and shea butter have been used for centuries for their skin-softening and smoothing properties, and are available in many different grades.

Cocoa butter is mainly used in the chocolate-making industry and therefore is very easy to find as food-grade or organic. The cosmetic grades tend to be refined and deodorized, because not everyone wants their cocoa-butter products to smell like chocolate. I love the smell myself so I tend to use food-grade or organic cocoa butter rather than the deodorized version. You can also buy a dark cocoa butter that smells strongly of chocolate, which is great in bath melts and chocolate-flavored lip balms but is not really suitable for body products due to the color.

There are many Fairtrade suppliers of shea butter that support the communities of the (usually) women who produce it. The unrefined/unfiltered shea does go off much faster than the filtered version, so unless you intend to use it within a few months it is best to buy it filtered. Adding an antioxidant to your finished product (such as vitamin E) will extend the shelf life.

TO USE

This rich, tropical-smelling body butter is best used after a bath or shower and massaged into slightly damp skin. It is very rich, so you don't need to use much, but do pay extra attention to areas such as elbows, knees, and feet, which are more prone to dryness. It's a great product to take on vacation and use in the evening after a day in the sun. You could use organic or food-grade solid coconut oil (non-deodorized) instead of the mango butter, or mix half and half for a really tropical smell.

Ingredients

10g beeswax or jojoba wax

25g cocoa butter

30g shea butter

25g mango butter

1 teaspoon (5ml) almond oil

1 teaspoon (5ml) vitamin E

10 drops lime essential oil

5 drops sweet orange essential oil

5 drops lemon essential oil

Equipment

double boiler

metal spoon

airtight 3½fl oz (100ml) jar

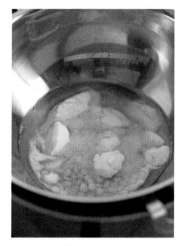

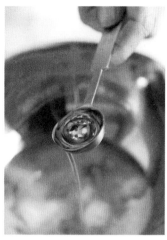

1 Melt the beeswax, cocoa butter, shea butter, and mango butter in the double boiler. If you have time, leave the mixture over a gentle heat for about 20 minutes, because this will help prevent the butter going grainy when it cools.

2 Add the almond oil and vitamin E and heat for a few more minutes until everything is liquid.

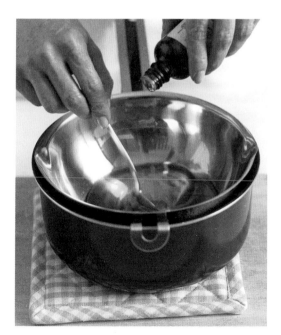

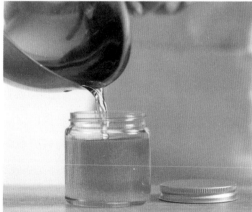

3 Remove from heat and add the essential oils, stirring thoroughly.

4 Carefully pour the warm mixture into the jar and leave to set.

Vetiver & vanilla body cream

You know there are some times when you just want to use a product that feels and smells gorgeous and luxurious; well this body cream is for those times. It is a very simple and straightforward recipe, but the combination of coconut, vetiver, and vanilla smells just divine. If you want to go all out, add some rose and patchouli to the mix!

If rose otto or absolute is stretching the budget a little too far, then replace the spring water with rosewater instead, and you could always use some almond oil that has been macerated with a vanilla pod instead of the vanilla extract (see p.122 for more information on how to do this).

Vanilla

Vanilla absolute smells very different to the sugary synthetic vanilla scents that you find in commercial bath and body products. However, it is quite difficult to work with due to its thick, treacle-like consistency, and its brown color can be a problem. It is hardly ever used nowadays in mainstream products, since it will turn white cream a brown color, and most consumers want vanilla-scented products to be snow white.

I love the CO2 extract of vanilla, which although still thick is much more mobile than the absolute. Do remember though that, as this is still a natural extract, your body cream will be a lovely cream color rather than pure white and may get darker over time.

Ingredients

Oil phase

10g coconut oil

5g shea butter

7g emulsifying wax

2 teaspoons (10ml) almond oil

1 teaspoon (5ml) macadamia oil

Water phase

4 tablespoons (60ml) spring water

½ teaspoon (2.5ml) glycerin

Cooling phase

10 drops vitamin E oil

20 drops preservative (or according to manufacturer's instructions)

10 drops vanilla absolute, or CO2 extract

5 drops vetiver essential oil

5 drops cedarwood essential oil

Equipment

double boiler

small glass jug

small saucepan

thermometer

electric (or battery-operated) milk frother (see equipment chapter) or stick blender

bowl of cold water

metal spoon

airtight 3½fl oz (100ml) jar

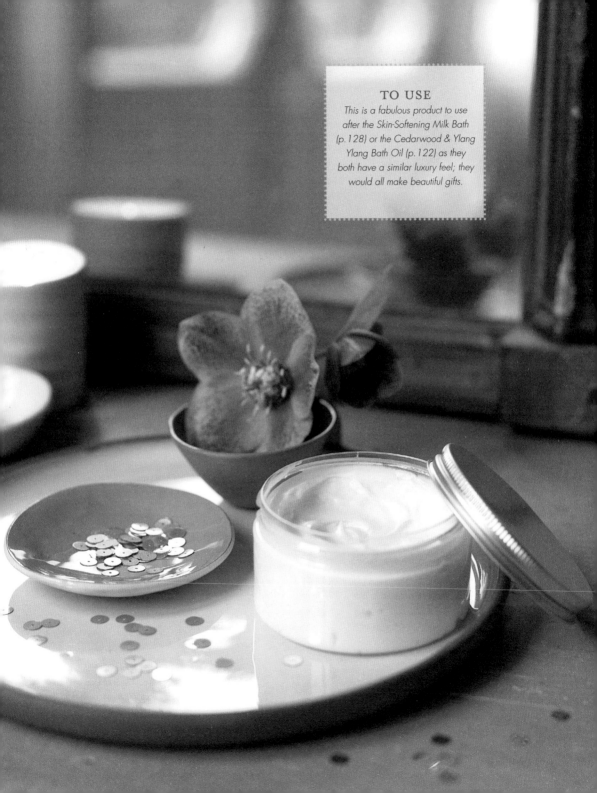

TO USE

This is a fabulous product to use
after the Skin-Softening Milk Bath
(p.128) or the Cedarwood & Ylang
Ylang Bath Oil (p.122) as they
both have a similar luxury feel; they
would all make beautiful gifts.

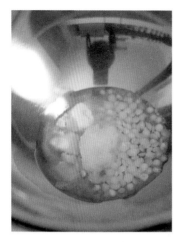

1 For the oil phase, melt the coconut oil and shea butter in the double boiler along with the emulsifying wax.

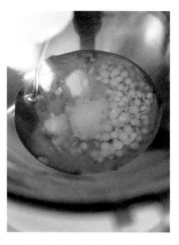

2 Add the almond and macadamia oils and heat until all is liquid.

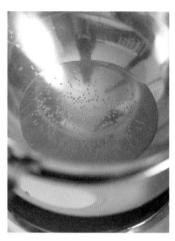

3 For the water phase, heat the spring water and glycerin in a glass jug placed in a saucepan of hot water, or using a second double boiler.

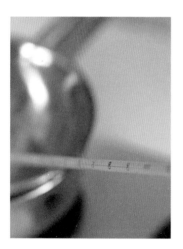

4 Heat until the oil phase ingredients have melted and both the oil and water phase have reached the same temperature of 167–176°F (75–80°C).

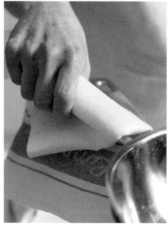

5 Remove the water phase from the saucepan of water, taking care not to burn yourself. Always hold with a cloth.

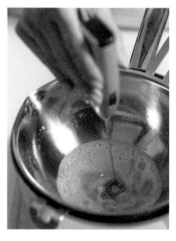

6 Place the milk frother or stick blender into the oil phase, which should still be in the double boiler. Turn on to a low setting, taking care to keep the blender in contact with the base of the pan so as not to introduce too much air into the cream.

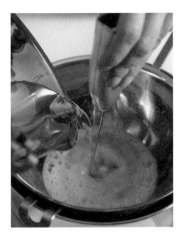

7 In a steady stream, pour the water phase into the oil phase while continually blending with the milk frother. Continue for approximately one minute.

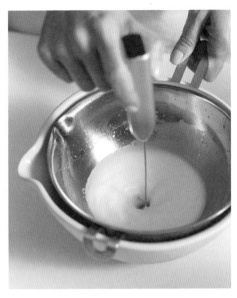

8 Place the double boiler containing the lotion into the bowl of cold water and continue to blend until the mixture thickens slightly.

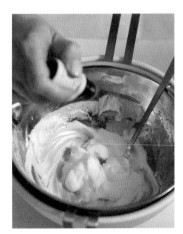

9 Once the mixture has cooled, stir in the vitamin E, preservative, and essential oils.

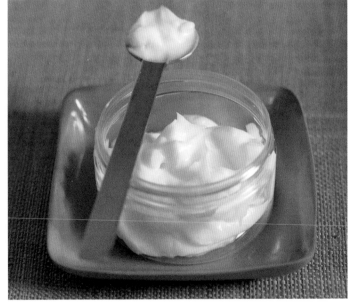

10 Pour into the jar. Make sure you label clearly with the date and ingredients used.

Barbados-ready body scrub

This body-scrub recipe was inspired by a friend of mine who shared a goal for the year, which was to be "Barbados Ready." Initially it meant losing a few pounds and being perfectly groomed with a capsule wardrobe that could be packed in an instant, should someone invite her to hop on a plane the next day to fly to Barbados.

As the year progressed, however, it came to mean much more than that, and it was an idea that was adopted by a group of us. We cleared all our clutter, both physically and mentally. We recycled belongings that we no longer needed to others who did, and we streamlined our lives, pledging not to acquire any more unnecessary "stuff." More importantly, we stepped back, took stock, and decided to take a bit more care of ourselves (which is where the scrub comes in!).

This may seem like an awful lot to ask of a body scrub, but if nothing else it will make your skin feel "Barbados Ready" and smell like a tropical cocktail.

Coconut oil

Pure coconut oil is a great body moisturizer. Although is solid at room temperature, it is soft enough to be easily rubbed into the skin. It can also be used as a pre-shampoo treatment for dry and damaged hair, and is sometimes referred to as coconut butter. I have also used macadamia oil, to fit in with the tropical theme and for its moisturizing properties, but you could replace it with almond oil. Sugar forms the exfoliating part of this recipe, and it is up to you which kind you use. The finer the sugar, the gentler the scrub will be; similarly, the chunkier the grains, the rougher it will be. I find demerara sugar works best for me, but experiment with different types until you find one you like best.

Ingredients

1¾oz (50g) coconut oil (solid)

2 teaspoons (10ml) macadamia oil

10 drops orange essential oil

5 drops lemon essential oil

5 drops lime essential oil

2oz (60g) raw (unrefined) brown sugar

Equipment

small glass bowl or mug

teaspoon

airtight 3½fl oz (100ml) jar

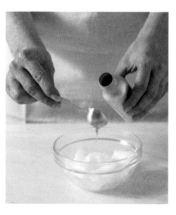

1 Add the coconut oil to the bowl or mug.

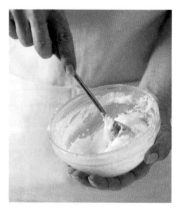

2 Add the macadamia oil to the mixture, then stir the oil and coconut mixture vigorously with a teaspoon, whipping it up until soft and fluffy.

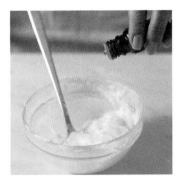

3 Add the essential oils and stir, ensuring they are evenly distributed in the mixture.

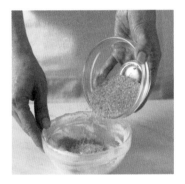

4 Add the brown sugar gradually to the coconut oil mixture, stirring carefully to ensure it is all mixed in.

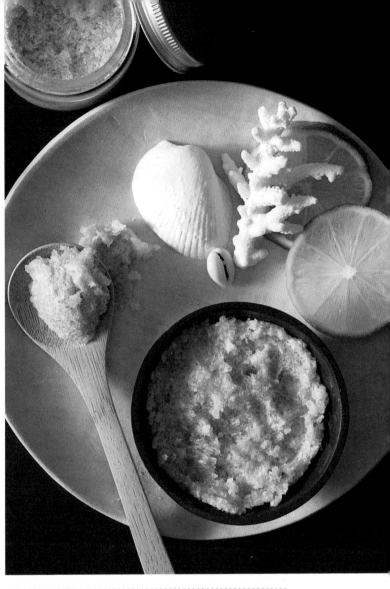

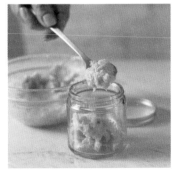

5 Carefully spoon the mixture into the jar.

TO USE

Massage into damp skin while in the shower, paying special attention to knees and elbows. Always go easy when using scrubs on the delicate skin on the collarbone and chest. Rinse off the scrub and you will be left with a layer of the coconut oil, which you can massage into your skin to keep it soft and supple.

Comfrey & arnica massage oil

This massage oil is great for after sports or any other physical exertion because it contains macerated oils, which help to alleviate aches, pains, and strains. Comfrey is included for healing bruises, strains, and sprains as well as helping to regenerate skin cells in sensitive or rough damaged skin.

St John's wort is anti-inflammatory, antiviral, and astringent. It is commonly used nowadays for treating anxiety and depression, but is also very useful for healing cuts and scrapes, soothing sensitive or itchy skin, and for rheumatism and back pain. Arnica is a well-known remedy for bruising, aches and pains, and sports injuries.

Add up to 2 percent of the total volume of your own blend of essential oil, depending on the properties you require. I have suggested two different blends for you to try.

Ingredients

2 teaspoons (10ml) comfrey oil

2 teaspoons (10ml arnica oil

2 teaspoons (10ml) St John's wort oil

4 teaspoons (20ml) avocado oil

1½fl oz (45ml) almond oil

1 teaspoon (5ml) vitamin E

approx. 20–40 drops essential oils:

Relaxing blend: 6 drops lavender, 6 drops geranium, 4 drops clary sage, 4 drops bergamot

Warming sports blend: 4 drops coriander, 2 drops ginger, 4 drops black pepper, 6 drops orange, 4 drops cedarwood

Equipment

small glass jug or beaker

metal spoon

airtight 3½fl oz (100ml) glass bottle

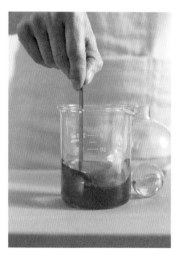

1 Add the oils, one at a time, to the glass jug, then add the vitamin E.

2 Add the essential oils and mix thoroughly. Pour into the glass bottle.

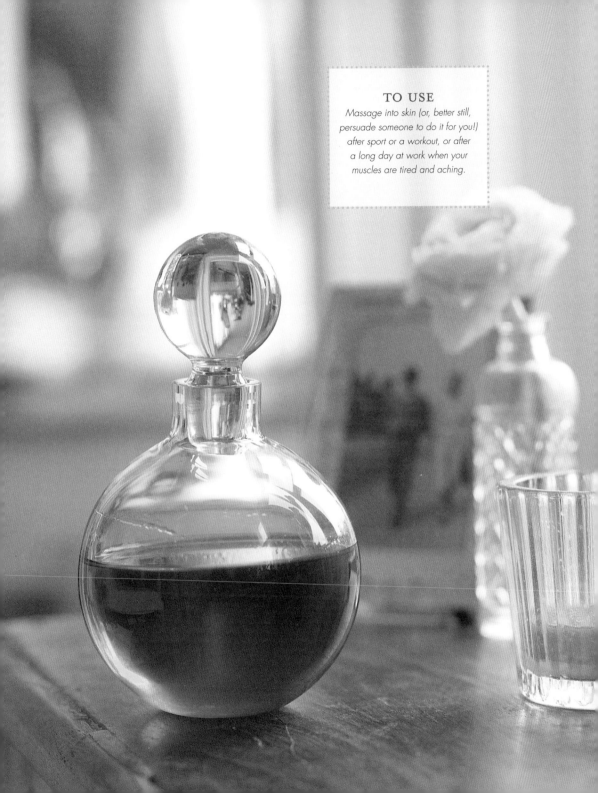

TO USE

Massage into skin (or, better still, persuade someone to do it for you!) after sport or a workout, or after a long day at work when your muscles are tired and aching.

Lavender & aloe vera body gel

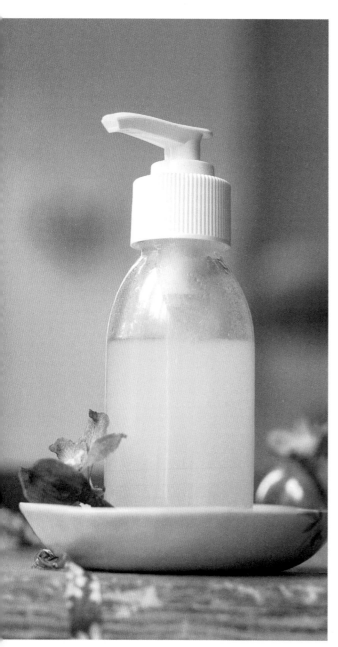

Aloe vera, which makes an excellent houseplant and is easy to grow indoors, is one of the best natural ingredients for soothing irritated or sunburned skin. Simply break off a leaf, strip off the outer green part, and apply the mucilage directly to the skin. You cannot, however, incorporate fresh aloe vera from the plant into skincare products unless you are going to use them straight away, as it goes bad very quickly. Most aloe vera that you buy is freeze-dried from the plant and then diluted to make a concentrate with some preservative added. This can then be incorporated into creams, lotions, and homemade gels. Gels are very easy to make at home using food-based gelling agents such as xanthan gum or the slightly more difficult to find konjac root powder.

Konjac glucomannan powder

Konjac glucomannan powder is from the root of the Asian plant *Amorphophallus konjac*, and it is used extensively as a diet aid and health supplement in pill or capsule form. Due to its fibrous nature, when added to water it forms a really solid gel structure and is amazing for creating easy eye, face, body, and anything else gels. I much prefer it to xanthan gum. I would suggest you try both and see which one you like best. The basic gel recipe can be adapted and also stirred into creams and lotions once they have cooled to add a lovely light and fluffy texture.

Ingredients

2 teaspoons (10ml) aloe vera concentrate

½ teaspoon (2.5ml) calendula oil

½ teaspoon (2.5ml) rosehip seed oil

3½fl oz (100ml) Basic Gel (see below and right), cooled

20 drops lavender essential oil

For the basic gel

½ teaspoon 2.5ml glycerin

20 drops preservative (or according to manufacturer's instructions)

2¾fl oz (85ml) spring water

1g konjac glucomannan powder or xanthan gum

Equipment

small glass jug

metal mixing spoon

whisk or stick blender

3½fl oz (100ml) bottle with pump dispenser

To make the basic gel (makes 3½fl oz/100ml)

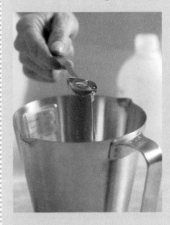

Add the glycerin and preservative to the jug.

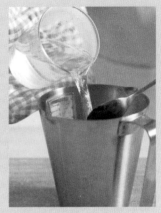

Bring the water to the boil, add to the jug, and stir the mixture to dissolve the ingredients.

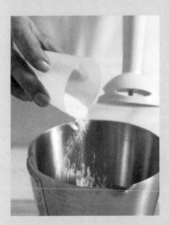

Sprinkle the konjac powder onto the boiling water.

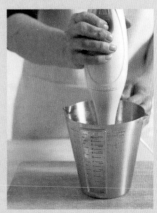

Whisk thoroughly until there are no lumps. Leave to cool before using.

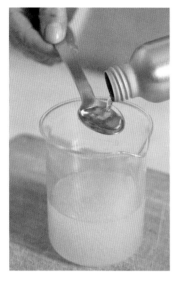

1 Stir the aloe vera concentrate, calendula oil, and rosehip seed oil carefully into the cooled basic gel.

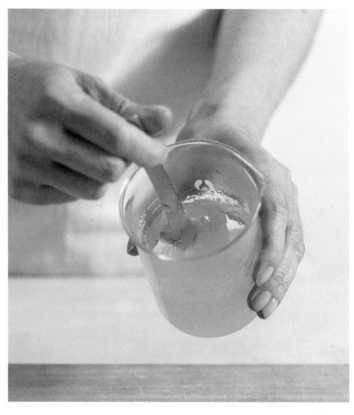

2 Add the lavender oil and stir gently to incorporate it thoroughly.

3 Carefully pour the mixture into the bottle.

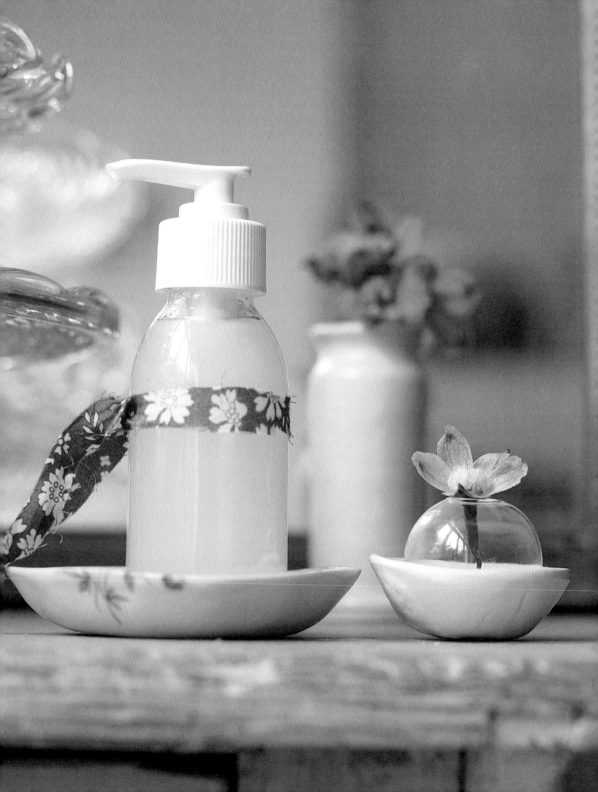

Shea butter & lemongrass hand softener

This hand cream has the amazing scent of lemongrass, which I love because it reminds me of Thailand and the gorgeous spas they have there, where its sweet, lemony, and warming scent is used as an insect repellent. I have used it in this recipe for its refreshing, deodorising, and antiseptic properties. St John's wort is often used as a natural antidepressant, but, when used topically in either oil or tincture form, it helps to heal cuts and scrapes.

As this cream contains water, a preservative should be added to prevent the growth of mold and bacteria. If you do not want to add a preservative, it will need to be kept in the refrigerator and will last a week at the most. I would suggest halving the amount so that you use it more quickly and using a small clean spoon when removing it from the jar to prevent contamination.

Ingredients

Oil phase

10g shea butter

2 teaspoons (10ml) almond oil

6g emulsifying wax

6g cetearyl alcohol)

Water phase

1¾fl oz (55ml) spring water

1 teaspoon (5ml) vegetable glycerin

Cooling phase

1 teaspoon (5ml) St John's wort oil

15 drops lemongrass essential oil

20 drops preservative (or according to the manufacturer's instructions)

Equipment

double boiler

small glass jug

small saucepan

electric (or battery-operated) milk frother (see equipment chapter) or stick blender

bowl of cold water

metal spoon

airtight 3½fl oz (100ml)jar

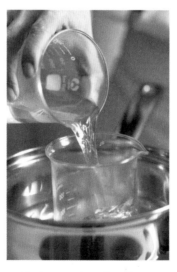

1 For the oil phase, add all the ingredients to the double boiler and heat until everything has melted.

2 For the water phase, heat the spring water and glycerin in a glass jug placed in a saucepan of hot water, or using a second double boiler.

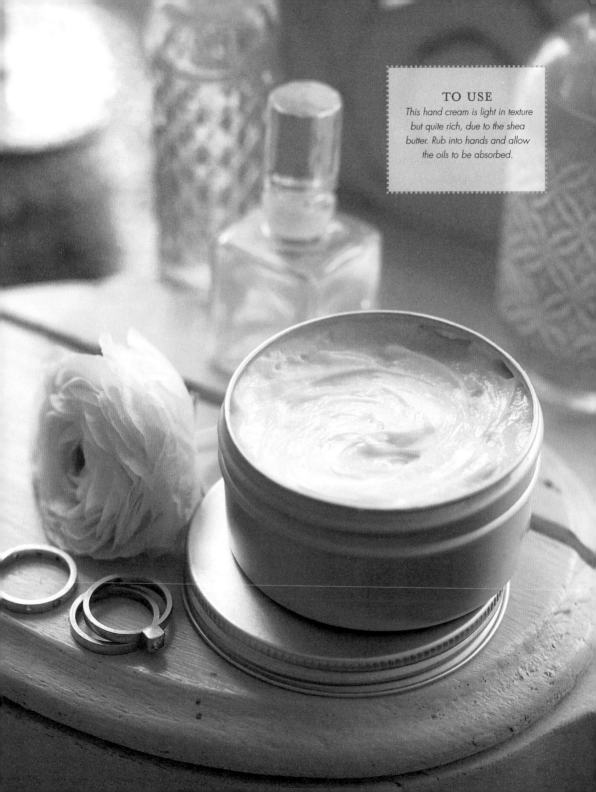

TO USE

*This hand cream is light in texture
but quite rich, due to the shea
butter. Rub into hands and allow
the oils to be absorbed.*

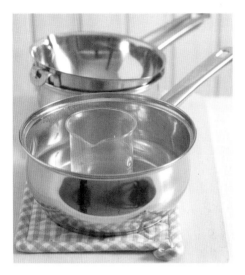

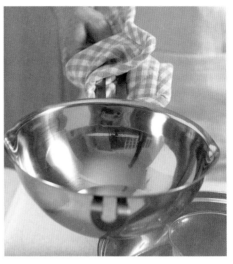

3 Once your oil phase and water phase have reached the same temperature of 167–176°F (75–80°C), remove both from the hob.

4 Remove the oil phase from the saucepan of water, taking care not to burn yourself. Always hold with a cloth.

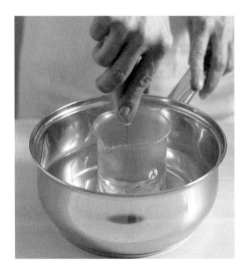

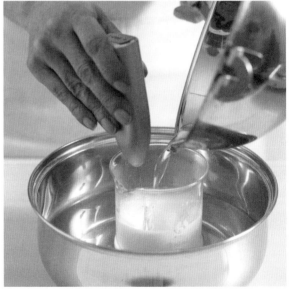

5 Place the milk frother or stick blender into the water phase, which should still be over or in the saucepan of hot water. Turn on to a low setting, taking care to keep the blender in contact with the base of the jug so as not to introduce any air into the cream.

6 In a steady stream, pour the oil phase into the water phase whilst continually blending with the milk frother. Continue for approximately one minute.

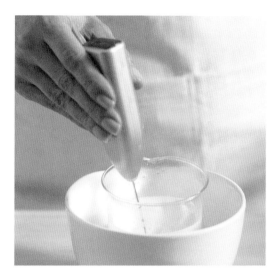

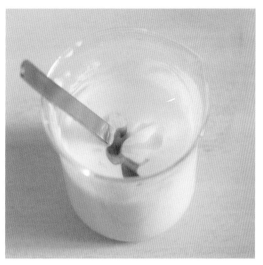

7 Place the jug containing the cream into the bowl of cold water. Continue to blend until the mixture thickens slightly.

8 Once the mixture has cooled, stir in the St John's wort oil, preservative, and essential oils.

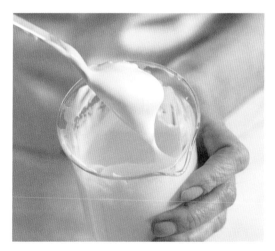

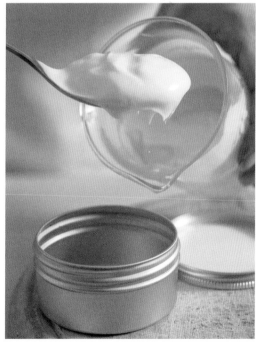

9 To help the thickening process, put the mixture in the refrigerator for a few minutes and then stir. Repeat until the mixture is thick.

10 Carefully spoon the mixture into the jar and label clearly with the date and ingredients used.

Rosemary & lemon handwash

Both rosemary and lemon essential oils have antibacterial properties as well as a lovely fresh smell that works well to remove any strong odors from the hands. The base recipe is very similar to a basic shower gel (as used in the Bergamot & Grapefruit Wake-up Wash, p.132), so you could, in fact, make up a large batch of base and customize with different essential oils and additives.

I have used a rosemary infusion as the water content because it goes with the theme of the recipe, but you could play around with different herbs, depending on your preference. You could use calendula or chamomile instead or chickweed infusion for sensitive itchy skin or a flower water such as lavender. I have included aloe vera for skin soothing and some glycerin, too, for its humectant properties.

To make the infusion

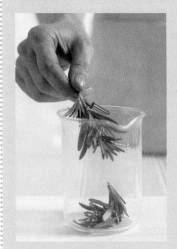

Place 5g fresh or dried rosemary in a mug or jug.

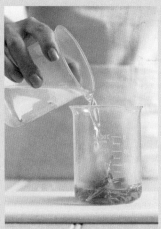

Pour on 3½fl oz (100ml) boiling spring water and leave covered for around 30 minutes.

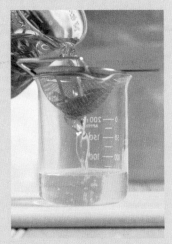

Pour the mixture through a tea strainer and discard the herbs. Use the infusion in your recipe. Any leftover infusion can be stored in the refrigerator for a couple of days.

Ingredients

3 tablespoons (45ml) natural surfactant blend, such as Plantapon (see ingredients section, p.23)

½ teaspoon (2.5ml) thickener/moisture-restoring agent, such as Lamesoft (see Glossary, p.142)

3 tablespoons (45ml) cooled rosemary infusion (see below left)

½ teaspoon (2.5ml) glycerin

1 teaspoon (5ml) aloe vera

20 drops preservative (or according to the manufacturer's instructions)

10 drops rosemary essential oil

10 drops lavender essential oil

20 drops lemon essential oil

10—40 drops lactic acid (to adjust pH to 5.5)

Equipment

2 small glass jugs

tea strainer

metal spoon

pH test strips

3½fl oz (100ml) bottle with pump dispenser

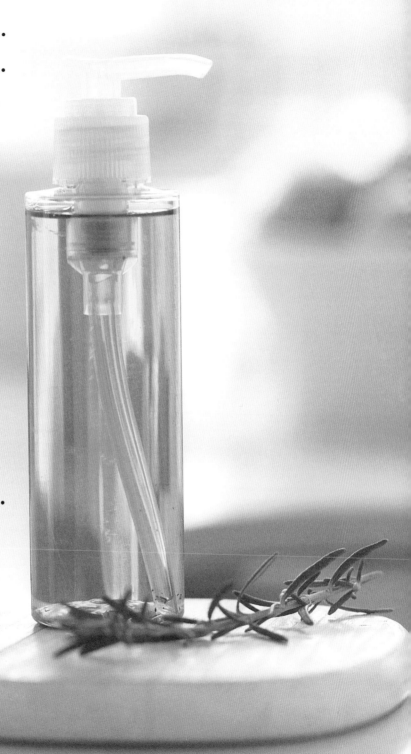

1 Spoon the Plantapon and Lamesoft
  into one of the jugs.

2 Pour the rosemary infusion into the
  other jug, add the glycerin and aloe
vera, and stir with a metal spoon.

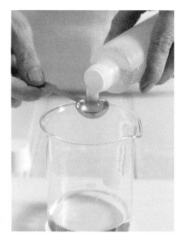

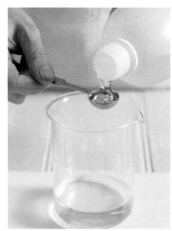

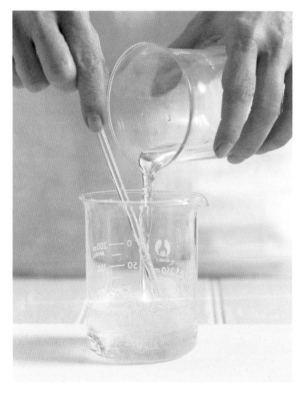

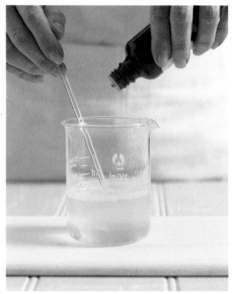

4 Add the preservative and essential oils, again mixing
  carefully so as not to create any foam.

3 Add the rosemary infusion to the Plantapon and Lamesoft mixture,
  stirring gently until they are all blended, but take care not to whip the
mixture and so cause foaming.

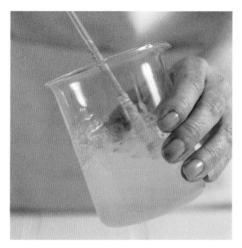

5 Dip a pH test strip into the mixture. If it registers above pH 5.5, add a few drops of lactic acid.

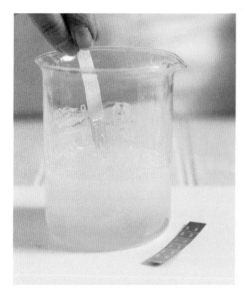

6 Retest and add more lactic acid a drop at a time until the mixture reaches the correct pH (when the gel will thicken).

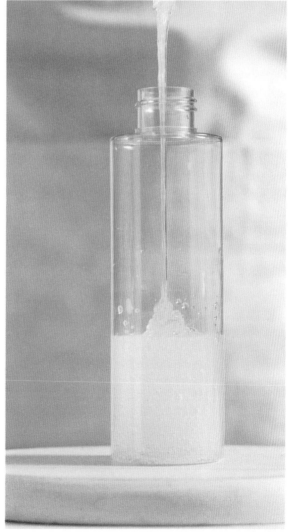

7 Pour into the bottle and label with the date and ingredients.

Pumice & peppermint foot scrub

Our feet are probably the most hard-working parts of the body, bearing our weight and carrying us around all day, but they are often the most neglected. For most of us, the only time we pay them any attention is when summer comes around and we have to expose them in all their dry, flaky glory, with just a hasty splash of nail polish to draw attention away from our cracked heels. However, the good news is that with regular attention during the winter months, come the summer it will be a different story.

It's quite easy to get away with using a thick, emulsifying wax-based cream here, as it will be rinsed off. You do need some kind of emulsifier, rather than making an oil and beeswax balm, otherwise it is difficult to wash the pumice off. You could also stir some pumice or apricot kernel powder into a gel base instead, as that will be fairly easy to rinse off, although mix up only a small amount to use immediately, as the pumice will sink to the bottom.

Pumice

Pumice is actually a type of solidified lava that occurs naturally in areas of volcanic activity and has been used for centuries for its abrasive exfoliating properties. It is far too abrasive for use on the face or body but is good for removing hard skin on the feet and is often used in heavy-duty hand cleansers. Peppermint essential oil is both cooling and refreshing, just what you need after a hard day on your feet. It is a very pungent essential oil that is used as a flavoring in the food industry and for toothpaste; only a few drops are needed for you to be able to feel its full effects.

Ingredients

Oil phase

5g cocoa butter

5g shea butter

7g emulsifying wax

2 teaspoons (10ml) almond oil

2 teaspoons (10ml) castor oil

Water phase

3 tablespoons plus 1 teaspoon (50ml) spring water or floral water (hydrolat) of your choice

1 teaspoon (5ml) glycerin

Cooling phase

20 drops preservative (or according to the manufacturer's instructions)

10 drops peppermint essential oil

10g pumice powder

Equipment

double boiler

metal spoon

small glass jug

small saucepan

thermometer

electric (or battery-operated) milk frother (see equipment chapter) or stick blender

bowl of cold water

airtight 3½fl oz (100ml) jar or bottle with pump dispenser

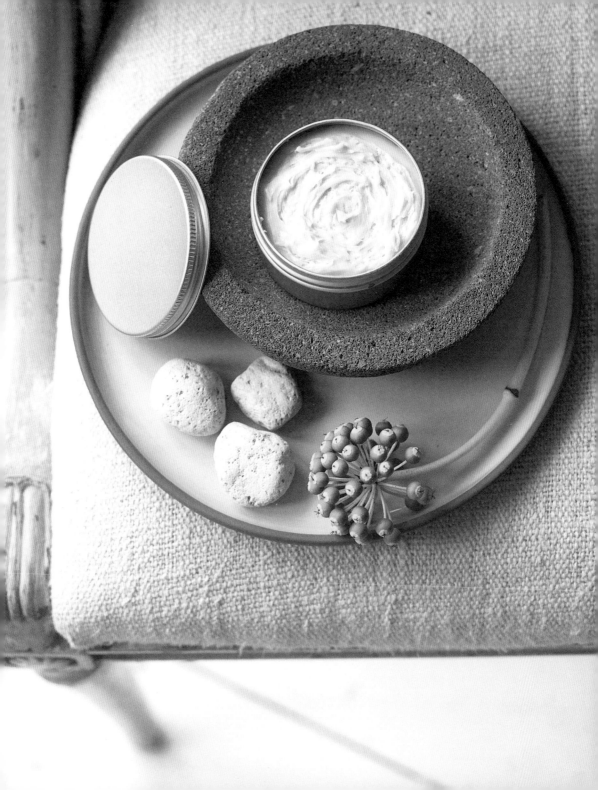

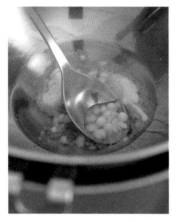

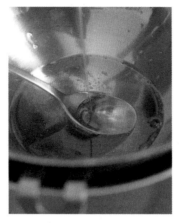

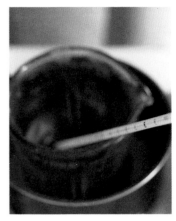

1 For the oil phase, melt the cocoa butter and shea butter in the double boiler along with the emulsifying wax.

2 Add the almond and castor oil and heat until all is liquid.

3 For the water phase, heat the spring water and glycerine in a glass jug placed in a saucepan of hot water, or using a second double boiler, until boiling. Heat until the oil phase ingredients have melted and both the oil and water phase have reached the same temperature of 167–176°F (75–80°C).

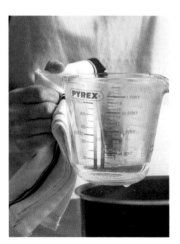

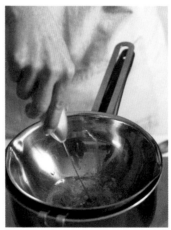

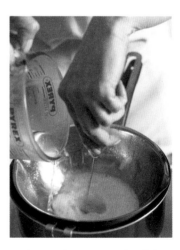

4 Remove the oil phase from the saucepan of water, taking care not to burn yourself. Always hold with a cloth.

5 Place the milk frother or stick blender into the water phase, which should still be in the jug in the pan of hot water. Turn to a low setting, keeping the blender in contact with the base of the jug so as not to introduce any air into the cream.

6 In a steady stream, pour the oil phase into the water phase while continually blending with the milk frother. Continue for approximately one minute.

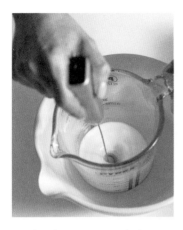

7 Place the jug containing the lotion into the bowl of cold water and continue to blend until the mixture thickens slightly.

8 Once the mixture has cooled, stir in the preservative, peppermint essential oil, and pumice powder gradually so that they are evenly dispersed throughout the cream. If you feel that the mixture is not scrubby enough, add a bit more pumice powder until you get the desired consistency.

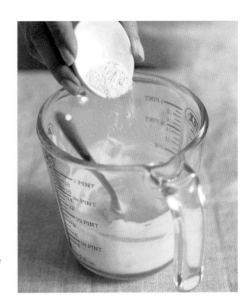

9 Spoon into the jar or bottle and label with the ingredients and the date.

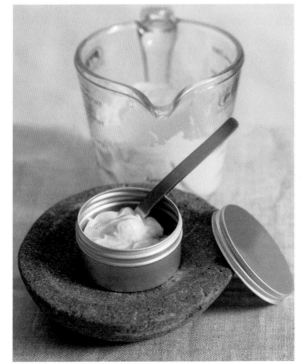

TO USE
Use this scrub as part of a pedicure, starting with a relaxing foot soak. Gently massage the scrub into your soles and heels, paying attention to the ends of the toes, which can also be prone to hard skin. Rinse thoroughly to remove any traces of pumice and dry with a warm soft towel. Apply Lemon & Tea Tree Foot Balm (see p.104) or Kokum Butter Foot Cream (see p.106) as a finishing touch.

Lemon & tea tree foot balm

The ingredients in this balm can be varied depending on the purpose you require it for. As it is, it makes a very rich and nourishing foot treatment for dry and cracked skin. I have used kokum butter, because it is excellent for softening really dry skin especially on feet, but you could replace it with shea butter instead if kokum butter is hard to find. The essential oils are both antiseptic and antibacterial as well as making your feet smell nice!

For cooling and refreshing, peppermint on its own works well or you could try mixing peppermint with lemon instead of the tea tree. Comfrey (*Symphytum officinalis*), historically known as "knitbone" or "boneset," is used in this recipe to encourage healing of cracked skin—it has a historical usage for mending broken bones. It contains a protein called allantoin, which helps with cell division and has soothing and anti-irritant properties.

Ingredients

15g beeswax

20g cocoa butter

2 tablespoons (30ml) almond oil

10g coconut/neem oil

2 teaspoons (10ml) comfrey oil

10g kokum butter (or shea butter)

1 teaspoon (5ml) Vitamin E

10 drops lemon oil

10 drops tea tree oil

Equipment
double boiler

metal spoon

airtight 3½fl oz (100ml) jar

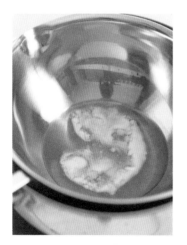

1 Melt the beeswax and cocoa butter in the double boiler.

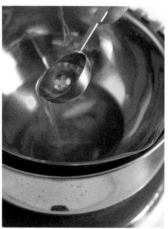

2 Add the almond oil and coconut oil (or neem) and stir gently with the spoon until everything is liquid.

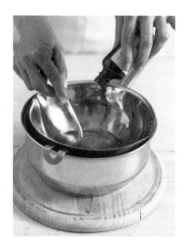

3 Remove from the heat and stir in the remaining ingredients, ensuring everything is completely blended.

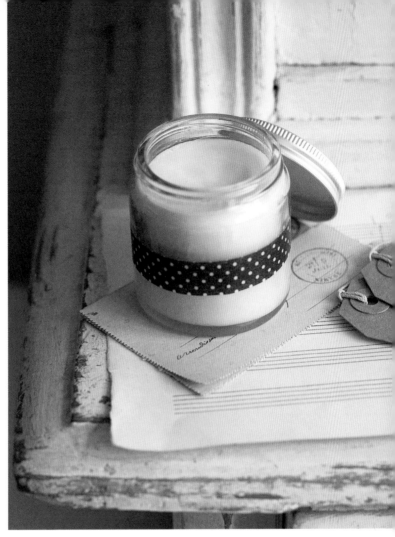

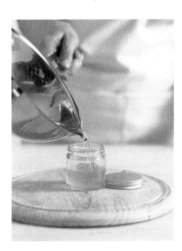

4 Carefully pour the mixture into the jar and leave to set.

VARIATION

If you suffer from athlete's foot, add 5 drops myrrh essential oil to the blend and replace the coconut oil with neem oil instead. Neem is an amazing antibacterial and antifungal oil but has a very strong characteristic odor, which some find unpleasant; it really is worth putting up with this for its effects though and the strong scent of the tea tree, lemon, and myrrh should go some way to masking it.

Kokum butter foot cream

Kokum butter is a very recent discovery for me. I tried it in a body cream recipe instead of cocoa butter and it gave the most amazing texture, which, although a bit too heavy for me as a body cream, works perfectly as either a hand or foot cream.

It has been traditionally used in India for its healing properties on dry, cracked, and calloused skin and for its ability to help regenerate the skin's cells. It is thought to help restore elasticity and flexibility of the skin and prevent dry skin and wrinkles. It is slightly softer and flakier than cocoa butter, so if you do not have any kokum and use cocoa butter instead, this will give the cream a slightly firmer texture but it is perfectly fine otherwise.

For the water phase of the cream, I use either peppermint or tea tree floral water (hydrolat), but you can use any other floral water that takes your fancy or an infusion made by pouring boiling water on a peppermint tea bag (although do make sure that there are no additives other than peppermint herb in the tea bags).

Ingredients

Oil phase

5g shea butter

10g kokum butter

6g emulsifying wax

2 teaspoons (10ml) almond oil

Water phase

4 tablespoons (60ml) tea tree or peppermint water (you could make a peppermint infusion or use plain spring water if you prefer)

1 teaspoon (5ml) glycerin

Cooling phase

20 drops vitamin E oil

20 drops preservative (or according to the manufacturer's instructions)

10 drops lemon essential oil

10 drops tea tree or peppermint essential oil

Equipment

double boiler

small glass jug

small saucepan

thermometer

electric (or battery-operated) milk frother (see equipment chapter) or stick blender

bowl of cold water

metal spoon

airtight 3½fl oz (100ml) jar

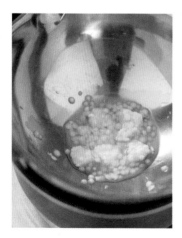

1 For the oil phase, melt the shea and kokum butters in the double boiler with the emulsifying wax.

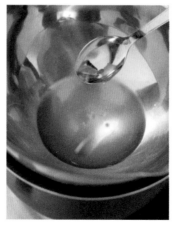

2 Add the almond oil and heat until all is liquid.

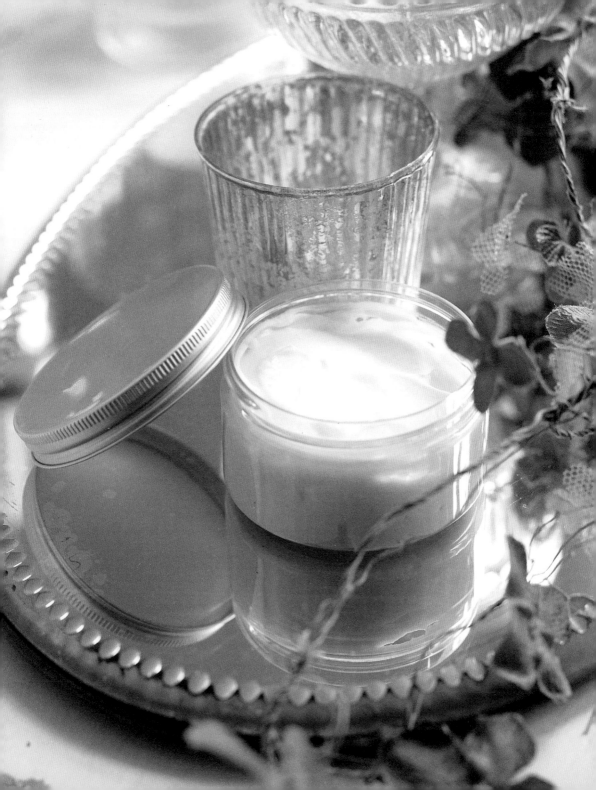

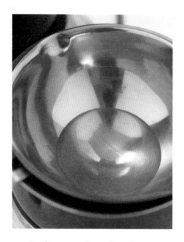

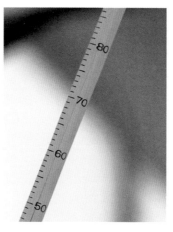

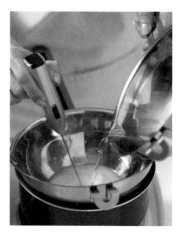

3 For the water phase, heat the tea tree or peppermint water and glycerin in a glass jug placed in a saucepan of hot water, or using a second double boiler.

4 Heat until the oil phase ingredients have melted and both the oil and water phase have reached the same temperature of 167–176°F (75–80°C). Remove the water phase from the saucepan of water, taking care not to burn yourself. Always hold with a cloth.

5 Place the milk frother or stick blender into the oil phase, which should still be in the double boiler. Turn on to a low setting, taking care to keep the blender in contact with the base of the pan so as not to introduce any air into the cream.

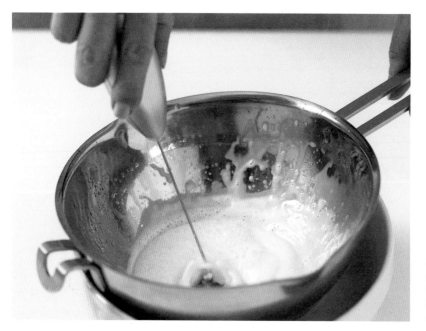

6 In a steady stream, pour the water phase into the oil phase while continually blending with the milk frother. Continue blending for approximately one minute.

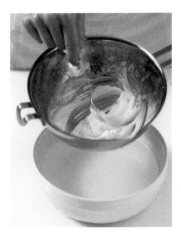

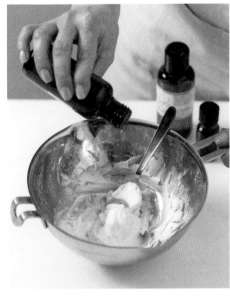

8 Once the mixture has cooled, stir in the vitamin E oil, preservative, and essential oils.

7 Place the double boiler containing the lotion into the bowl of cold water and continue to blend until the mixture thickens slightly.

9 Pour or spoon into the jar. Make sure you label clearly with the date and ingredients used.

TO USE

Massage into dry cracked skin on feet, hands, and elbows. You can vary the flower water and essential oils you use depending on preference. Lemon, peppermint, and tea tree are great for feet, but you may wish to use something a bit more gentle and less pungent if you intend to use it on other parts of the body.

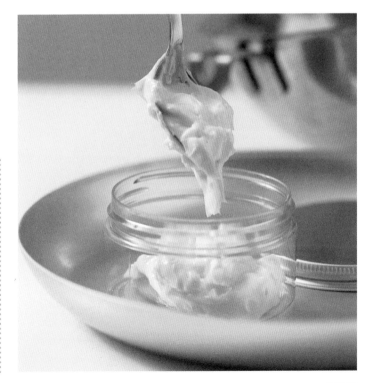

Geranium & orange massage bars

Essentially, a massage bar is a solid version of a massage oil and is very eco friendly as it needs no packaging. It is a good idea, though, to keep them wrapped and in the refrigerator, as they are prone to melting in hot weather and do gather dust if left unwrapped.

The base is very simple, and if you use cocoa butter as the main ingredient you do not need to add beeswax to hold it together. Cocoa butter is a fabulous ingredient that melts on contact with the skin and is great to use during pregnancy on areas prone to stretch marks to keep them supple.

This recipe makes two 2oz (50g) bars; you can easily scale up the quantities and make extras as gifts. You may need to check the volume of the molds you are using and adjust the quantities accordingly, as different molds will vary.

Ingredients

2½oz (70g) cocoa butter

1oz (30g) shea butter

10 drops orange essential oil

10 drops geranium essential oil

Equipment

double boiler

plastic soap molds or silicone muffin molds

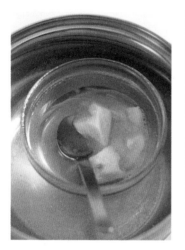 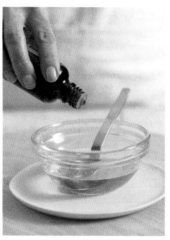 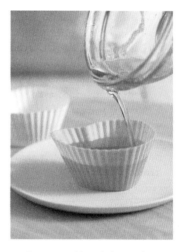

1 Melt the cocoa butter and shea butter in the double boiler, or in a bowl over a pan of boiling water.

2 Remove from the heat and add the essential oils.

3 Pour into molds and place in the refrigerator to set.

TO USE
Massage into the skin as a moisturizer after a bath or shower.

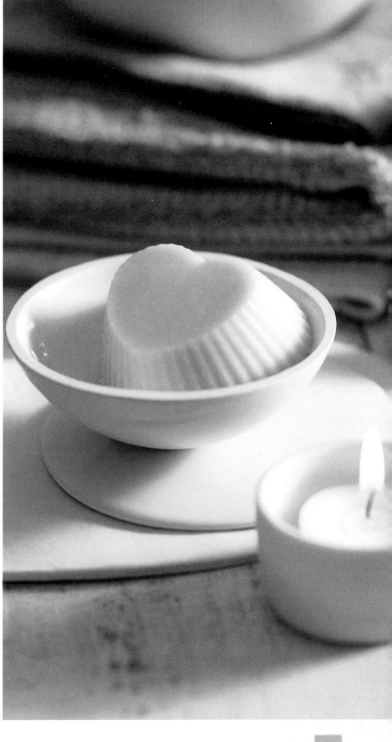

Choosing molds

These make great gifts,
and you can use your
imagination when it comes
to molds. Make mini ones
in ice-cube trays or look
in cookware shops for
chocolate bar or mini
egg molds.

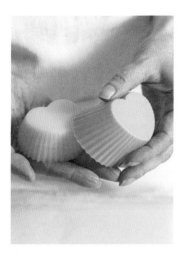

4 Once the bars have set, remove from
the molds and wrap in either foil or
greaseproof paper to keep them clean.

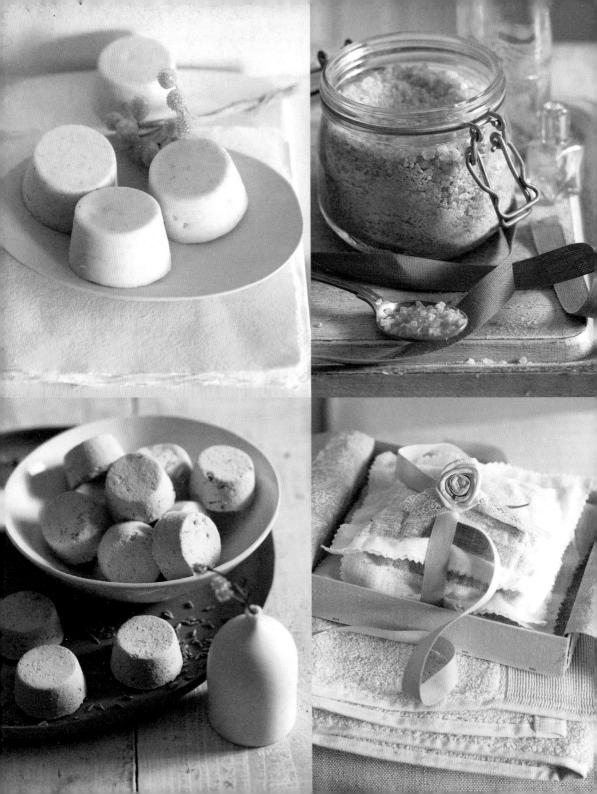

chapter 4

Bath and shower

Relaxing in a long, hot bath is one of life's luxuries
we very seldom make time for, so use the recipes in
this chapter as an excuse for a bit of pampering. Take
some time out and create your own deliciously scented
bath products—they are wonderfully simple to make, and
I have even included a shower gel recipe for those of you
too busy to relax in the bath. If you prefer a traditional
approach to bathing, then making your own soap is
the way to go as long as you follow the safety rules
and don't mind waiting several weeks for it to cure.
The results are well worth the wait!

Mint-choc bath melts

Bath melts can be made with regular cocoa butter, but if you use the dark organic unrefined grade, they look like chocolates and make a great low-calorie alternative gift. Do make sure you put a "do not eat" warning on them, though, as they do look and smell like the real thing. You could leave out the essential oils if you want plain chocolate, or mint works well, as does sweet orange. Feel free to experiment with blends such as geranium and orange or rose otto for an indulgent Turkish delight scent. You could make these in mini guest soap or chocolate molds, silicone ice-cube trays in various shapes, or mini fondant cases.

Ingredients

3½oz (100g) dark cocoa butter

3 tablespoons plus 1 teaspoon (50ml) almond oil

20 drops peppermint essential oil

Equipment
double boiler

chocolate molds or ice-cube tray

kitchen foil or an airtight jar

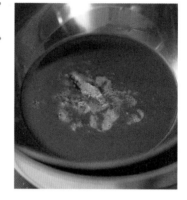

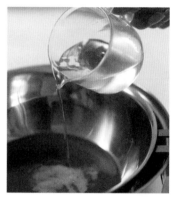

1 Melt the cocoa butter in the double boiler, or in a bowl over a pan of boiling water.

2 Remove from the heat and add the almond and essential oils.

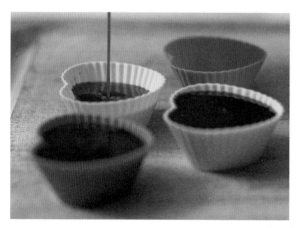

3 Pour into the molds and leave to cool, then place in the refrigerator to set. Once the mixture has set, remove from the molds. Either wrap in foil or store in an airtight jar.

TO USE
Just drop one or two into a hot bath.

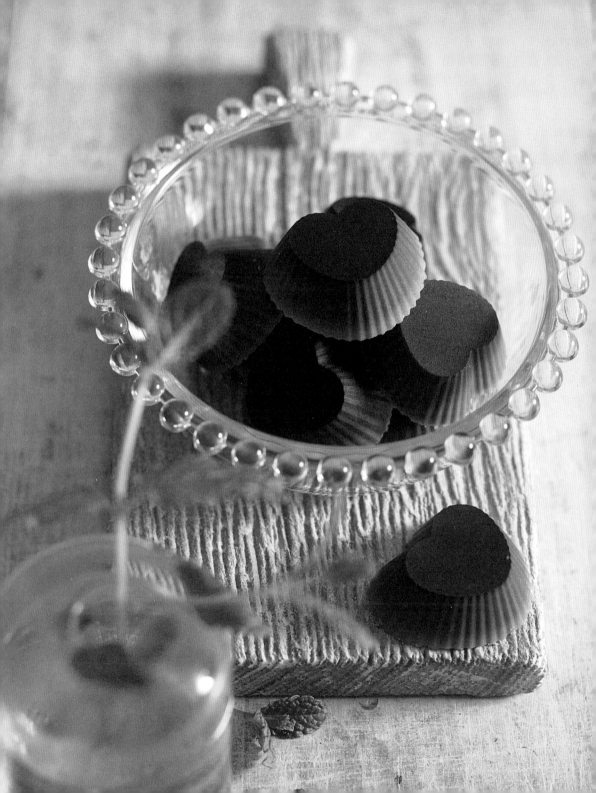

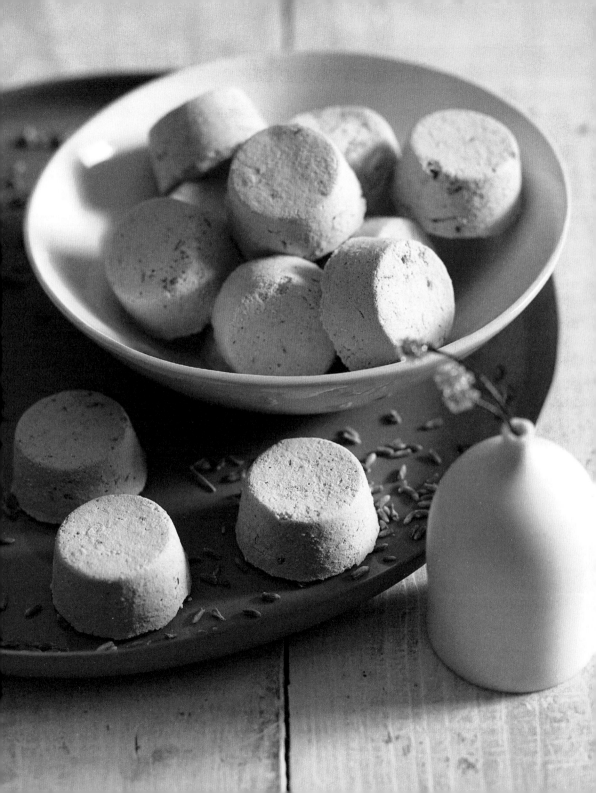

Lavender & clary sage bath fizzes

One of my favorite relaxing bath blends is lavender and clary sage. When dropped into running water, these bath fizzes fill the air with their gorgeous aromatic herbal scent.

Lavender is very well known for its healing and relaxing properties, and many people use it topically for burns, cuts, scrapes, and spots. It is also used in many commercial toiletries.

Clary sage, however, is less frequently used, but it is very effective for helping to calm and relax the nerves, sending you off into a deep sleep if used before bedtime. Clary sage is also useful for helping to alleviate menstrual pain, either by adding it to a bath or diluting it in a vegetable-oil base and massaging it over the abdomen. Clary sage should not be used during pregnancy, nor should it be used when drinking alcohol, due to its soporific effect.

Ingredients

5¼oz (150g) sodium bicarbonate

2¾oz (75g) citric acid

1oz (25g) cornstarch (cornflour)

½ teaspoon powder color or 2 drops liquid color (optional)

10 drops clary sage essential oil

15 drops lavender essential oil

1 tablespoon dried lavender flowers

spray bottle of witch hazel or water

Equipment

sifter (sieve)

mixing bowl

silicone muffin molds

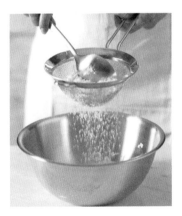 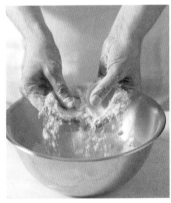 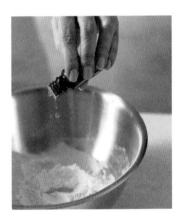

1 Sift the sodium bicarbonate, citric acid, and cornstarch into a bowl, and mix thoroughly.

2 Add the powder or liquid color and blend into the mixture until there are no lumps. This is usually best done with your hands, rubbing the mixture between your thumb and fingers as if you were making pastry.

3 Add the essential oils and rub in again until the fragrance is totally blended in. You can wear latex (or non-latex) gloves to protect your hands from the neat essential oils. Add the lavender flowers, if using.

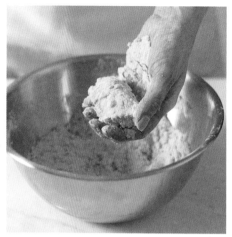

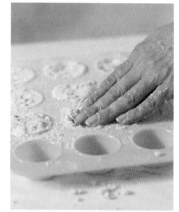

5 Take a handful of the mixture and pack it tightly into each mold, pushing the mixture in as firmly as possible. The tighter you pack it in, the better the result will be. Repeat until you have filled all of the molds.

4 Take the spray bottle of witch hazel and spray the mixture several times while mixing with the other hand. Keep doing this until the mixture is the texture of damp sand. Be patient, adding the witch hazel gradually, and after each sequence of sprays squeeze a handful of mixture and drop it back into the bowl. When it holds its shape, it is ready to be packed into molds.

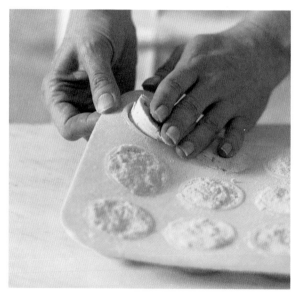

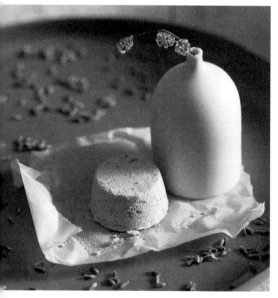

6 Leave the bath fizzes to harden overnight in a warm dry place before removing from the molds.

TO USE

Depending on the size of the molds you used, drop one or two into hot running water and relax in the bath.

Variation: Round bath bombs

If you are feeling more adventurous and would like to make a round bath bomb, you will need special molds that come in two halves. They are very easy to find online (see the suppliers listed on p.143). Round bath bombs are a little trickier to get right, though, and practice makes perfect. Follow the instructions for the bath fizzes up to the point of molding, and then proceed as follows.

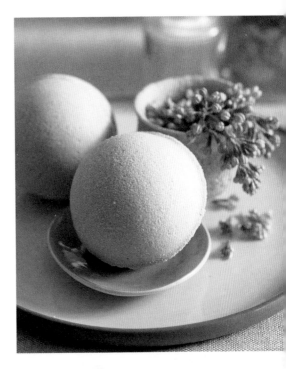

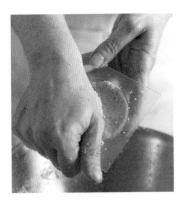

1 Take a handful of mixture and pack it tightly into each half of the mold, slightly overfilling one half.

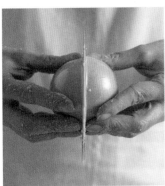

2 Push the two halves together (ensuring that they line up) for 20 seconds and then remove the top half of the mold. Dust off the excess mixture back into the bowl and leave the bath bomb to set.

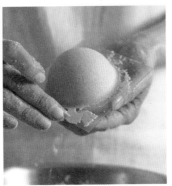

3 Repeat until you have filled all of the molds, working quickly so that the mixture does not dry out.

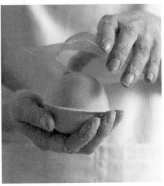

4 Carefully remove each bath bomb from the other half of its mold and place in a warm dry place to harden. To use, drop into hot running water.

Dead Sea detox bathing salts

With today's busy lifestyle, it probably isn't that often that you get half an hour to yourself to sink into a relaxing bath, and nowadays it is considered a luxury rather than a necessity. For personal hygiene, the majority of us quickly jump in and out of the shower before we go about our day; few people, I would imagine, take the time to bathe and contemplate the day ahead.

For the Romans and the Ancient Egyptians before them, however, it was a different matter: bathing was done for health and beauty reasons rather than just cleanliness, and these reasons were responsible for the popularity of spas. In fact, Cleopatra herself was reputed to have built the first day spa at the edge of the Dead Sea after hearing of the beautifying properties of the minerals therein.

Ingredients

6oz (175g) Dead Sea salt

6oz (175g) Epsom salts

4oz (150g) sea salt

2oz (60g) sodium bicarbonate

2oz (60g) powdered kelp or
green clay

30 drops juniper essential oil

20 drops fennel essential oil

20 drops lemon essential oil

30 drops grapefruit essential oil

Equipment

mixing bowl

metal spoon

airtight 2-cup (500ml) jar

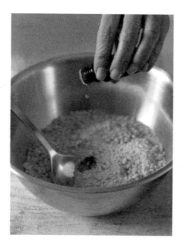

2 Mix thoroughly so that the salts and the powdered kelp or green clay are evenly distributed. Add your essential oils, stirring thoroughly with the spoon.

1 Put all the dry ingredients into the mixing bowl.

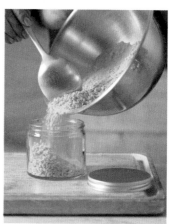

3 Pour into the jar and leave to sit overnight so that the essential oils infuse the mixture.

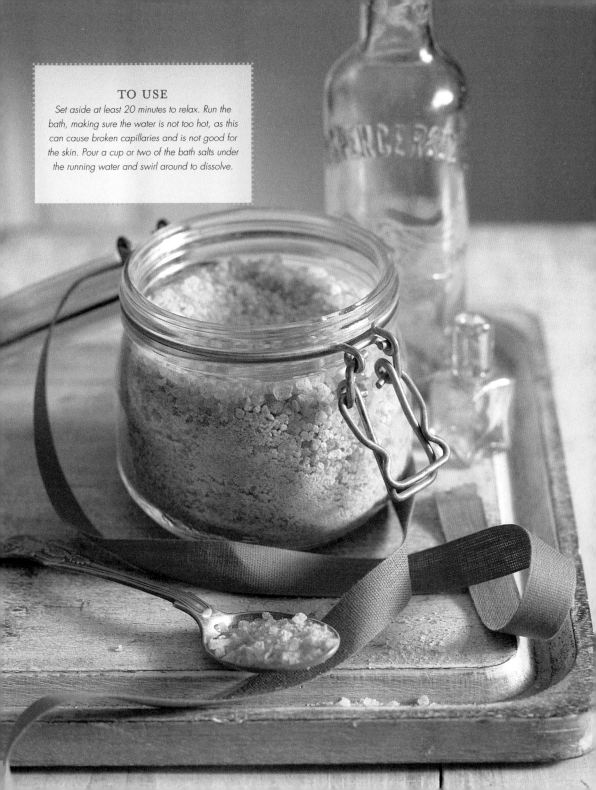

TO USE

Set aside at least 20 minutes to relax. Run the bath, making sure the water is not too hot, as this can cause broken capillaries and is not good for the skin. Pour a cup or two of the bath salts under the running water and swirl around to dissolve.

Cedarwood & ylang ylang bath oil

The essential oils in this bath oil were chosen for their gorgeous, heady, and exotic fragrances as well as their relaxing properties. Vanilla absolute or CO2 extract is delicious but quite expensive, so instead you could make your own vanilla-scented oil by placing a vanilla pod in some almond or jojoba oil for a few weeks to macerate. You can then use this as a base for making your own perfume oil or add it to your bath and body oil blends (removing the pod before using).

Ylang Ylang (*Cananga odorata*) oil is used in Indonesian wedding ceremonies for its aphrodisiac effects as well as in aromatherapy for its calming and sedative properties. Its sweet and heady aroma can be a bit overpowering if used in large amounts, so blend with other oils and use in small doses.

Ingredients

⅓ cup (80ml) sweet almond oil

4 teaspoons (20ml) apricot kernel oil

7 drops ylang ylang oil

6 drops cedar oil

3 drops geranium oil

4 drops orange oil

2 drops vanilla absolute or CO2 extract (or 2 tsp/10ml homemade vanilla-scented oil)

Equipment
small glass jug or beaker

metal spoon

airtight 3½fl oz (100ml) glass bottle

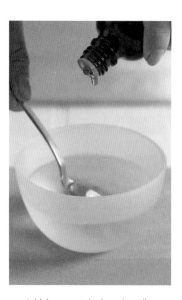

1 Add the sweet almond oil and apricot kernel oil to the glass jug or beaker.

2 Add the essential oils and vanilla absolute and mix thoroughly with the spoon. Pour into the glass bottle.

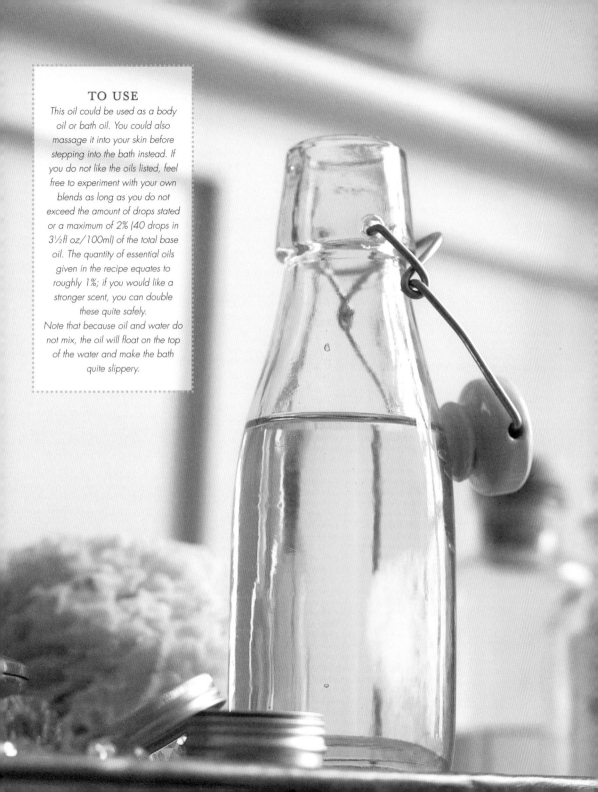

TO USE

This oil could be used as a body oil or bath oil. You could also massage it into your skin before stepping into the bath instead. If you do not like the oils listed, feel free to experiment with your own blends as long as you do not exceed the amount of drops stated or a maximum of 2% (40 drops in 3½fl oz/100ml) of the total base oil. The quantity of essential oils given in the recipe equates to roughly 1%; if you would like a stronger scent, you can double these quite safely.

Note that because oil and water do not mix, the oil will float on the top of the water and make the bath quite slippery.

Variation: Perfume oil

Most fragrances available today are a combination of natural and synthetic fragrance ingredients diluted in perfumer's alcohol, which, if you want to make your own fragrances, is impossible to buy over the counter in most countries without a license. As there are more independent artisans now making fragrance, we have seen a bit of a resurgence in both oil-based and solid perfume—harking back to the practices of the Ancient Egyptians.

Although perfumery is outside the scope of this book it is one of my passions, so I felt I had to sneak it in somewhere. When writing the recipe for Cedarwood & Ylang Ylang Bath Oil on the previous page, I actually created the fragrance blend first in 2 teaspoons (10ml) of jojoba oil to make sure it smelled good, before diluting it in 3½fl oz (100ml) of bath oil base. In fact, I would advise you to do this too when experimenting with blends in case they don't work out, because it saves wasting a lot of base oil.

Here is the recipe to turn the fragrance for the bath oil into both an oil-based and a solid perfume, which can be stored in either a lip balm tin or antique trinket or pill box.

Ingredients

2 teaspoons (10ml) jojoba oil

7 drops ylang ylang oil

6 drops cedar oil

3 drops geranium oil

4 drops orange oil

2 drops vanilla abstract or CO2 (or use jojoba that has been macerating with a vanilla pod)

Equipment

airtight ½fl oz (15ml) glass bottle

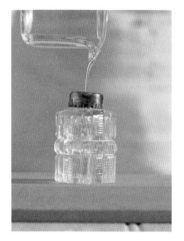

1 First pour the jojoba oil into the glass bottle.

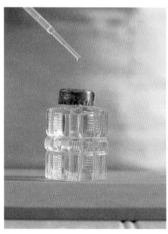

2 Add the drops of essential oils carefully.

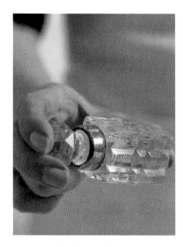

3 Place the lid on the bottle and shake to ensure all the oils are blended.

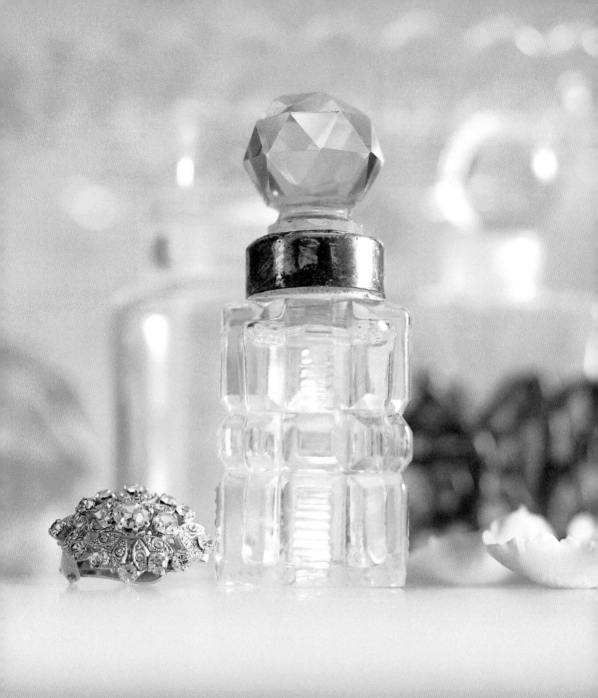

Variation: Solid perfume

For this variation I have doubled the quantity of essential oils, as I have doubled the base material. Since you are working with a small amount of material, it is best to use small heatproof container in a pan of simmering water to melt the beeswax rather than a double boiler.

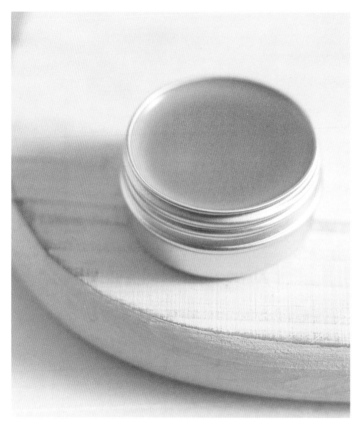

Ingredients

5g beeswax

3 teaspoons (15ml) jojoba oil

14 drops ylang ylang oil

12 drops cedar oil

6 drops geranium oil

8 drops orange oil

4 drops vanilla absolute or Co2
(or use jojoba that has been
macerating with a vanilla pod)

Equipment

small bowl, jug, or heatproof glass

shallow saucepan

small glass or egg cup

metal spoon

½fl oz (15ml) lip balm jar, tin,
or pretty pill box

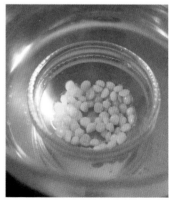

1 Melt the beeswax in a heatproof container placed in a shallow saucepan of boiling water.

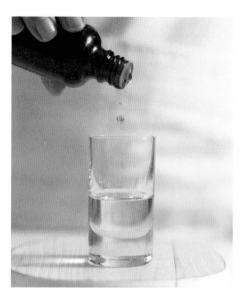

2 Measure the jojoba oil into a small glass or egg cup and add the essential oils.

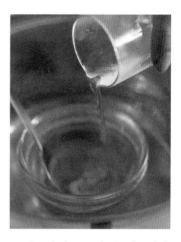

3 Once the beeswax has totally melted, carefully stir in the essential oil and jojoba blend.

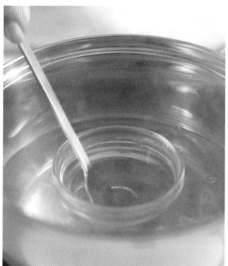

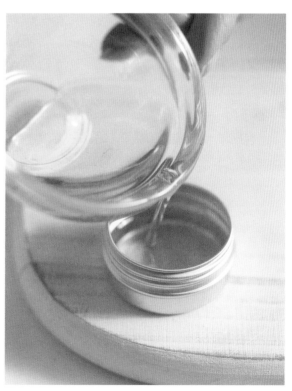

4 As heating will cause essential oils to evaporate, do not leave on the heat for very long—just until everything is liquid.

5 Remove from the heat immediately and pour into your chosen container. Leave the perfume to set.

Skin-softening milk bath

This is one of the very first recipes I ever made as a teenager and it is still one of my favorites. I had probably been reading about Cleopatra and her supposed beauty regime, and decided that I, too, should be bathing in asses' milk and rose petals!

If you are a vegan, you could make the same recipe with more sodium bicarbonate, or use kaolin (white clay) instead, but I love the luxuriousness that the milk powder gives. The cocoa butter melts in hot bath water and has a lovely moisturizing effect. The rose petals do look lovely in the jar but are not so lovely once wet, so they are more for decoration—don't use too many. Because the powdered ingredients take up so much space, this recipe will fill a 12fl oz (350ml) jar, even though the weight is only 5½oz (160g).

The longer you leave the vanilla pod in the jar, the stronger the scent will be, and the pod can be reused for subsequent jars. Make sure you remove it before giving this as a gift or before you tip the powder into a bath. I think vanilla works really well with goats' milk powder in products, and you could just store a vanilla pod in your jar or bag of milk powder so it is already impregnated with the scent for whenever you want to use it. If you don't like vanilla or do not have a vanilla pod, you could use essential oils instead.

Ingredients

1 vanilla pod (optional)

1¾oz (50g) goats' milk powder

3½oz (100g) sodium bicarbonate

20 drops essential oils (optional)

10g cocoa butter

handful dried red rose petals (optional)

Equipment

mixing bowl

metal spoon

cheese grater

airtight 1½-cup (350ml) jar

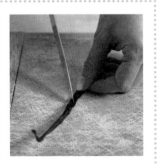

If you haven't stored your goats' milk powder with the vanilla pod already—and you want the scent of vanilla rather than using essential oils—score the pod gently with a sharp knife to let out the aroma and place in the jar.

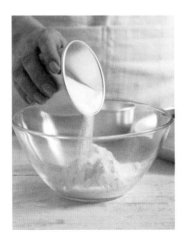

1 Place the vanilla-scented goats' milk powder and the sodium bicarbonate in the mixing bowl. Add the essential oils at this stage, if using, and mix thoroughly with the spoon.

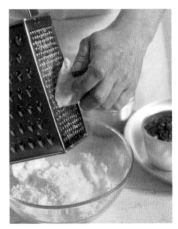

2 Grate the cocoa butter into the bowl, stirring in gently.

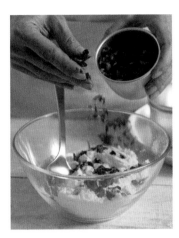

3 Stir through most of the rose petals. Sprinkle a few spoonfuls of the mixture into a running bath yourself (if you don't have any handmaidens to do it for you!).

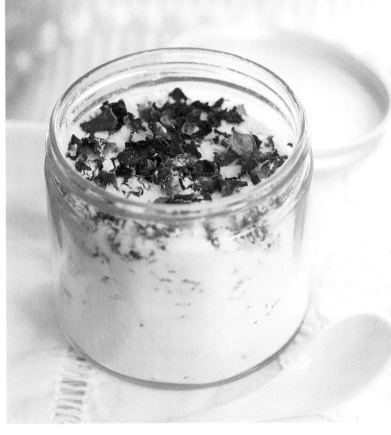

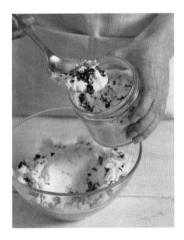

4 Spoon the remaining mixture into the jar. Sprinkle a few more petals on top for decoration.

Suggested essential oils

This recipe calls for all-out luxury, so choose sensual woods or heady floral oils that work with the milky scent of the goats' milk powder, such as ylang ylang, cedarwood, sandalwood, rose, geranium, patchouli, and vetiver.

Grating cocoa butter

Place the cocoa butter in the refrigerator (or freezer) before grating, since it will melt in your hands quite quickly. Use the finest side of the grater, so that you get a powder rather than chunks, and use either a pastry brush or a clean paintbrush to dust off any cocoa butter that sticks to the grater into the bowl, as it will melt if you use your fingers.

Herbal bath bags

I love to use fresh or dried herbs whenever possible in my bath and body products. In an ideal world, we would all be growing our own herbs in a beautifully manicured or naturally wild herb garden. If you are a keen gardener and have the space, it would be fabulous to have your own beauty garden filled with anything your local climate will allow to use in your homemade products. If, however, like me, you have no time, talent, or inclination for gardening, using dried herbs or liquid extracts is fine.

The easiest way to use dried herbs in the bath is with a traditional muslin bath sachet, which prevents the soggy herbs clogging up the plughole or sticking to your skin. Emerging relaxed and serene from a delicious herbal bath but covered in bits of soggy leaf and twig is not a good look!

Ingredients

For each bag you will need:

1 tablespoon of your chosen herb mix (see below) or just 1 or 2 herbs mixed together

Purifying herbs: rosemary, nettle, fennel, lavender, rock salt, seaweed

Relaxing herbs: chamomile, jasmine, hops, valerian, meadowsweet

Skin-soothing herbs: chamomile, oats, calendula, marshmallow, chickweed

Equipment

jar or bowl

approx. 8in (20cm) square of muslin

pinking shears

elastic band (not essential but so much easier than trying to tie a ribbon with one hand!)

length of narrow ribbon or natural twine, or a strip of muslin

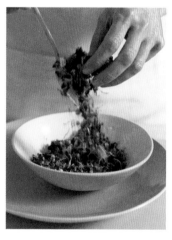

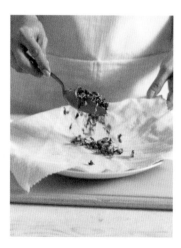

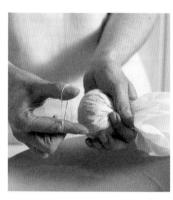

1 Mix the herbs together in a glass jar or bowl using equal parts of each herb.

2 Cut a muslin square with pinking shears and place a tablespoon of the mixture in the middle.

3 Place the elastic band over your thumb and forefinger and gather up the muslin into a pouch.

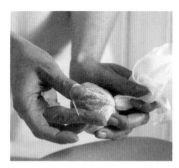

4 Secure the herbs inside with the elastic band, twisting and wrapping it several times.

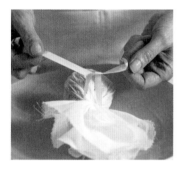

5 Tie with ribbon, twine, or muslin to hide the elastic band.

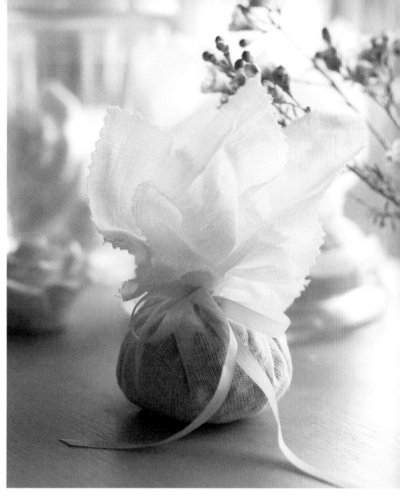

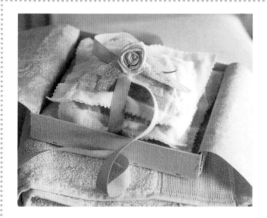

VARIATION

Bath bags also make very inexpensive but luxurious-looking gifts. Use some to fill a glass storage jar or place a few in a gift box tied with a ribbon.

If you are handy with a sewing machine, you could cut squares of muslin approximately 3½–4in (8–10cm) square with pinking shears so they look like ravioli. Sew along three sides, fill with the herbs, then sew the final side closed.

Bergamot & grapefruit wake-up wash

Making a basic shower gel is quite a simple process and it will give you an insight into what goes into products that we use every day and take for granted. Ultimately, there is no ingredient out there that doesn't have some degree of processing or effect on the environment—it is part and parcel of our 21st-century lifestyle and we just have to do the best we can to lessen our impact. There are many detergents that are used by large companies that are also available to the home crafter, and the best of the current bunch are listed on p.142.

The main components of a shower gel are detergent and water, which makes organic certification a bit of a gray area, since neither can be justifiably called "organic" (in the sense that we use the word today). Some companies get around this by including organic flower waters or water infused with organic herbs. The detergent blend used here is approved by EcoCert and is very easy to use in shower gels, shampoos, and liquid handwash. The other bonus with this ingredient is that no heating is involved in the recipe.

As detergents can be drying on the skin, we need to add a blend of coco glucoside and glycerol oleate to help prevent this, which will also act as a thickener for the shower gel. The key thing with this detergent blend is that it thickens automatically once the pH is 5.5 or less, so the lactic acid is important too.

Using preservatives

With such a large water content, which contains herbal extracts, a shower gel should be preserved to stop it becoming contaminated with bacteria—especially as it will be kept in a warm, damp, steamy environment. I have used a preservative that is effective only when the pH of the product is 5.5 or under, so have added a few drops of lactic acid to adjust it. Unfortunately, the preservative I have used for the creams and lotions is not effective in detergent bases, so we need to use a different one here. I realize that you may be using a slightly different preservative blend and advise getting directions from the supplier to make sure it is compatible with this recipe.

Ingredients

2 tablespoons plus 2 teaspoons (40ml) natural surfactant blend, such as Plantapon (see ingredients section, p.23)

½ teaspoon (2.5ml) thickener/ moisture-restoring agent, such as Lamesoft (see Glossary, p.142)

1 teaspoon (5ml) glycerin

3 tablespoons plus 1 teaspoon (50ml) orange flower water

20 drops bergamot essential oil

20 drops grapefruit essential oil

20 drops preservative (or according to the manufacturer's instructions)

10–40 drops lactic acid (to adjust the pH to 5.5)

Equipment

2 small jugs or bowls

metal spoon

pH test strips

3½fl oz (100ml) airtight plastic bottle

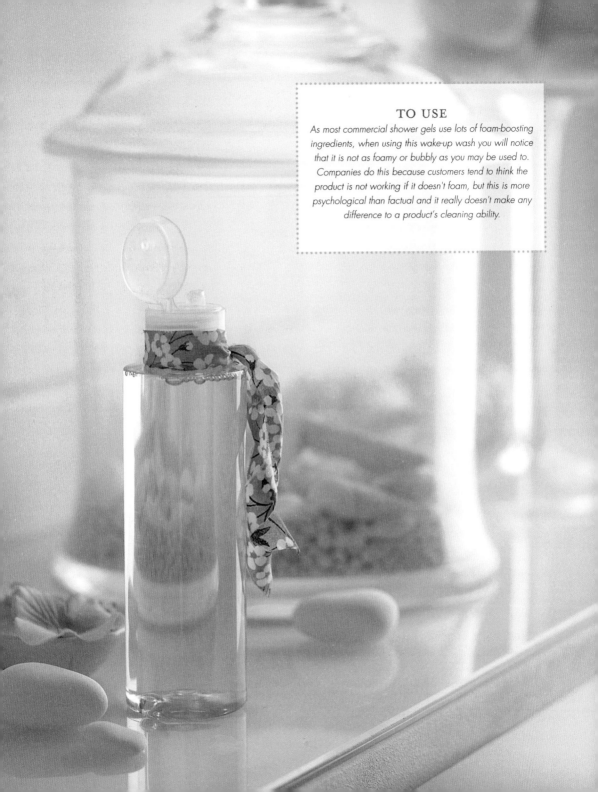

TO USE

As most commercial shower gels use lots of foam-boosting ingredients, when using this wake-up wash you will notice that it is not as foamy or bubbly as you may be used to. Companies do this because customers tend to think the product is not working if it doesn't foam, but this is more psychological than factual and it really doesn't make any difference to a product's cleaning ability.

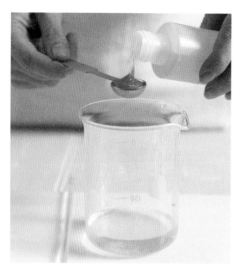

1 Measure the Plantapon and Lamesoft into one of the small jugs.

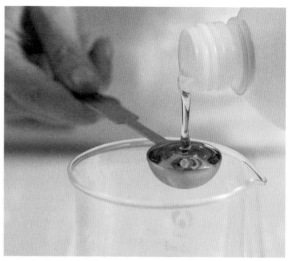

2 Measure the glycerin and orange flower water into the other jug and stir well with a metal spoon.

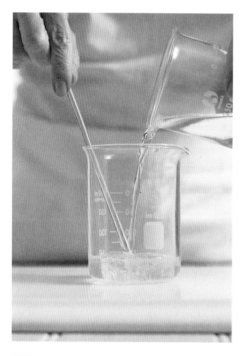

3 Pour the glycerin and orange flower mixture into the detergents, stirring gently until they are all blended, while taking care to not whip up and cause foaming.

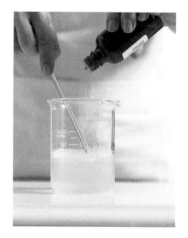

4 Add the essential oils and preservative, again mixing carefully so as not to create any foam.

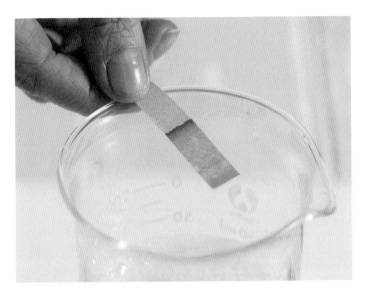

5 Take a pH strip and dip into the mixture. If it registers above pH 5.5, add a few drops of lactic acid.

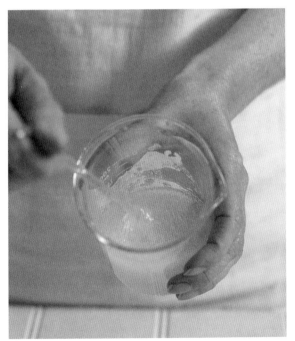

6 Retest, and add more lactic acid, a drop at a time, until the mixture reaches the correct pH (when the gel will thicken).

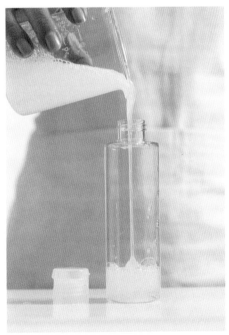

7 Pour into the bottle and label with the date and ingredients.

Handmade soap

The humble bar of soap is something most of us use on a daily basis without really thinking about where it comes from or what we are really using. Things have changed quite a lot in the soap industry over the last 50 years or so, and the chances are what you are using today is very different to what your parents or grandparents would have used. Much of the bar soap on the market nowadays is made from solid detergent rather than the saponified oils and fats that our ancestors would have used.

Soap is created by a chemical reaction between an alkali (sodium hydroxide, also known as caustic soda or lye) and an acid (oils or fats). Traditionally, animal fat would have been used, but this has fallen out of favor for obvious reasons. Coconut, olive, and palm oils are now widely used, especially by small companies selling handmade cold-processed soap bars. When the two are mixed together, a reaction called saponification takes place. This is where the alkali (lye/sodium hydroxide) reacts with the oils and fats to create soap and glycerin. Full saponification takes four to six weeks depending on the oils and fats used, which is why the soap can still be quite caustic until fully cured. Once the full curing time is up, all of the sodium hydroxide would have reacted with the oils and no longer be present as a separate entity.

Saponification

Different oils each have an individual saponification number, which tells you how much sodium hydroxide is needed to cause the saponification reaction to take place. There are

THE RULES OF SOAP MAKING

1. Treat sodium hydroxide with respect and store in a sealed container away from children and pets.
2. Always wear rubber gloves (with no holes) and safety goggles (not just spectacles) when using sodium hydroxide or handling freshly made uncured soap.
3. Always work in a well-ventilated area away from pets and children.
4. Always add sodium hydroxide to water—never the other way around—as the mixture can foam up. Always wear a facemask and goggles to protect yourself from the fumes; they last only a few moments.
5. Never touch your skin or rub your eyes with your gloves on. This may sound obvious, but both actions are easily done.
6. Keep a bottle of vinegar to hand in case any sodium hydroxide splashes on to your skin. If this happens, pour vinegar over it immediately, then rinse with cold water. If any sodium hydroxide gets into your eyes (which should never happen; you should be wearing safety glasses), rinse with cold water and seek immediate medical help. It can cause permanent eye damage, so make sure this never happens.

7. MOST IMPORTANT: Never, ever leave your soap mixture or sodium hydroxide unattended, or where children or pets can reach it—not even for a split second. If you hurt yourself by not following the rules, then it is your own fault. Your children and pets are your responsibility—keep them safe!
8. Use a stainless-steel pan (not nonstick or aluminum, as it will corrode) that is kept solely for soap making.
9. Weigh all the ingredients carefully because accuracy is very important.
10. Run all recipes through a SAP calculator (available online—see p.143) just to be on the safe side, especially if you make any changes to the oils used.
11. Do not use your soap until the full curing period is up as it will still be caustic.
12. Never, ever, break these rules!

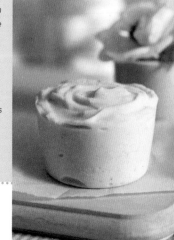

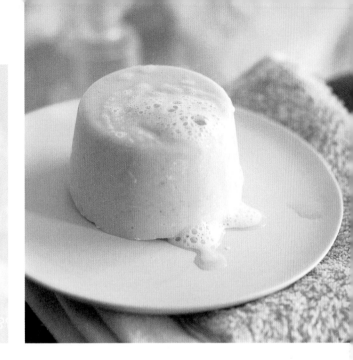

Commercial soaps

Commercial bar soaps are much harder and longer lasting than handmade bars, as they will have had the glycerin removed during processing. Handmade bars have a higher glycerin content and can be super fatted, which makes them much less drying on the skin. However, they will dissolve quicker, so they should be stored in a soap dish with a drainer to make them last a bit longer. "Super fatting" simply means that a percentage of the oil in your soap is not saponified but left free to add its moisturizing qualities to the soap.

a great many resources available online, including free saponification charts and calculators, to guide you through this process safely as well as many books specifically on the subject (see p.143).

Before you try out any cold-process soap recipes (including the one overleaf), it is always best to run the ingredients through a saponification calculator or at least become familiar with the values of the different oils, as even a minute change in the recipe can change the results—especially if you are converting grams to ounces or vice versa.

The trace stage

When reading through the method for a cold-process soap recipe, you will notice that you mix the combined oil and lye mixture until it reaches something called "trace." The length of time a soap batch takes to trace will depend on the oils used, as some take much longer than others; mixing with a stick blender rather than with a spoon by hand will speed up this process. Make sure you keep the blender in contact with the base of the pot and that your pot is big enough to prevent the mixture splashing, as it is still caustic at this stage.

As you stir the mixture, it will start to thicken until you can dribble a small amount of the mixture on the surface of the batch without it sinking. When this happens you have reached

trace, and essential oils and any colorants can now be added. If you add fragrances before this point, it may cause the batch to separate or curdle. If you are adding a powder color or clay, mix it with a small amount of water first. When adding fragrance to your recipe, be aware that any essential oils will be affected by the lye solution and potentially lose their therapeutic properties—so use the cheapest grade available as anything else will be a waste.

Soap safety issues

Many people (including me, for many years!) are put off making soap because mixing caustic soda with water and hot fat can be very hazardous if not done properly and following the correct precautions. When caustic soda is added to water, it will heat up naturally without any external heat source and create fumes that should not be breathed in. For this reason, you need to wear safety goggles and a facemask as protection, and work in a well-ventilated area.

It is a very simple and straightforward process but, just like driving a car, if you do not follow the rules and use utmost commonsense, you or your loved ones could face serious injury or even death. There are many true horror stories involving even experienced soap-makers. Please read the rules on the left carefully, word for word, at least ten times and imprint them in your brain before making soap.

Olive, coconut & sunflower soap

This is a very simple recipe to get you started, and I have chosen olive, sunflower, and coconut oils because they are all quite inexpensive and easy to obtain. The coconut oil is the same solid oil used in many of the skincare recipes in this book, while the sunflower oil is the type used for cooking. Olive oil is available in many grades; the grade that is best for soap-making purposes is known as olive pomace oil—which, luckily, is the cheapest grade available. Make sure it is pure olive pomace, as sometimes it is blended with other oils. A blended oil will have a different saponification value, which affects the amount of lye needed.

Please ensure that you weigh all the ingredients on a kitchen scale, including the liquids (which are given in grams for this purpose), because a high degree of accuracy is important. Essential oils and colors added at trace (see p.137) can be measured by volume as they will not affect the saponification process (see p.136).

I have used turmeric powder in this recipe to create a nice sunny orange color, along with sweet orange essential oil.

Before you start

1. Write out your recipe clearly on a piece of paper, and use this as a reference to tick off each ingredient as it goes into the pot, so that nothing gets missed out.

2. Set out your working area, which should be well ventilated, ensuring you have a supply of paper towels and vinegar near the sink.

3. Put on safety goggles, a safety mask, an apron, and rubber gloves.

4. Make sure you will not be disturbed as you work.

5. Re-read the safety rules on p.136.

Ingredients

400g coconut oil

400g sunflower oil

200g olive oil

330g water

150g sodium hydroxide

3–4 teaspoons (15–20ml) of a mixture of orange and lime essential oils

I teaspoon (5ml) ground turmeric

Equipment

rubber gloves, safety goggles, and face mask

vinegar (for first aid)

plastic jugs or bowls (for weighing ingredients)

large stainless-steel cooking pot

glass heatproof jug

metal spoon

muffin molds or plastic containers lined with parchment paper

sugar thermometer

stick blender

plastic spatula

plastic wrap (clingfilm)

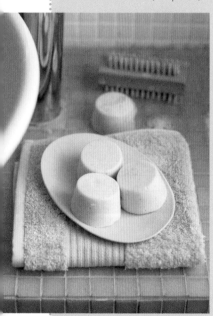

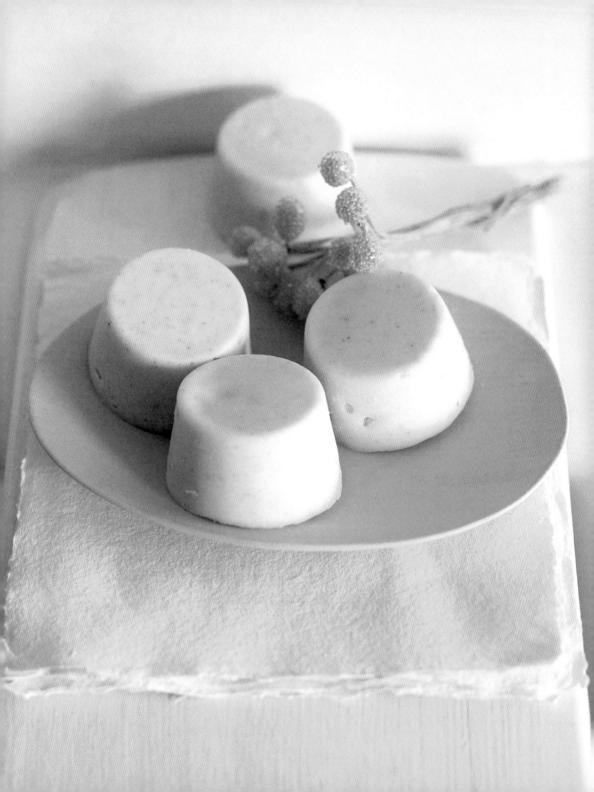

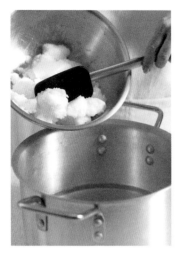

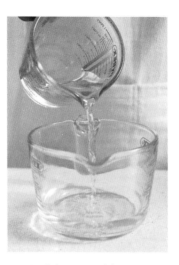

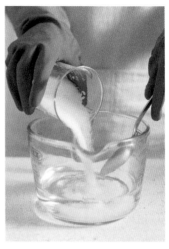

1 Weigh the coconut, sunflower, and olive oils and pour into the cooking pot, ticking off each as it is added.

2 Weigh the water and then pour it into the glass jug.

3 In a well-ventilated area, carefully add the sodium hydroxide to the water (not the other way round). Stir thoroughly, keeping your face away from the fumes.

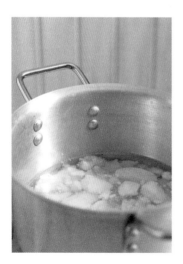

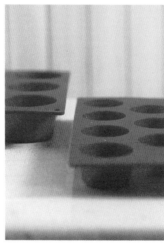

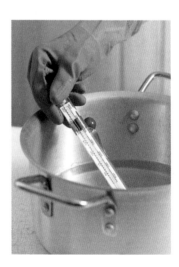

4 Melt the oils over a low heat; turn off the heat once melted.

5 Line your molds (if using silicone muffin pans, skip this step as they come out very easily).

6 Using the thermometer, check the temperature of the oils and the caustic soda solution until both reach 130°F (54°C).

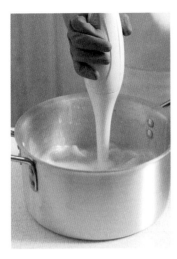

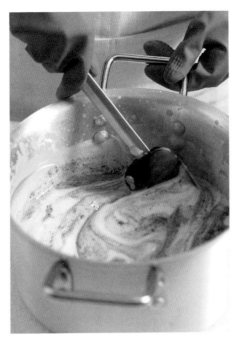

8 Add the turmeric or your chosen colorant, as well as clays or essential oils, and stir thoroughly.

7 Pour the caustic-soda solution into the fats, stirring carefully. Mix with the stick blender until the mixture reaches trace (when a dribble of mixture sits on the surface without sinking).

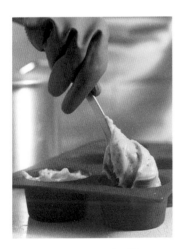

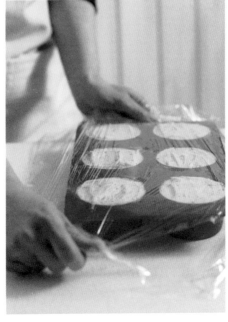

10 If you are using a plastic container and would like to cut the soap into bars, you should be able to do this approximately 48 hours later, or when set. Leave the soap to cure in a warm, dry place for at least four to six weeks before using.

9 Pour into the prepared molds, cover with plastic wrap (clingfilm) and leave to set in a warm, dry place. You should be able to remove the soap from the molds after 24 hours.

Glossary

Emulsifiers

GLYCERYL STEARATE A food-grade emulsifier derived from glycerin with stearic acid (a fatty acid obtained from either animal fats or vegetable oil—check with your supplier that their supply is from a vegetable source). It is used with other emulsifiers such as sodium stearoyl lactate and cetyl alcohol or cetearyl alcohol. Some companies in the US sell it ready mixed under a variety of trademarked names.

GLYCERYL STEARATE SE Also called glyceryl monostearate, this is "self-emulsifying" so does not need an extra emulsifier added. It can be used on its own with cetyl alcohol or cetearyl alcohol as a thickener. In a 3½oz (100g) recipe replacing 5g of emulsifying wax with 5g of glyceryl stearate SE, with the addition of 2–3g of cetyl alcohol, works well.

SODIUM STEROYL LACTATE A food-grade emulsifier that works in conjunction with glyceryl stearate. It is water soluble and derived from vegetable-source fatty acids plus lactic acid from bio fermentation.

CETEARYL GLUCOSIDE This combination of glucose and cetearyl alcohol is frequently used by natural skincare companies. It is a little tricky to use when making small quantities of lotion as the lotion will not thicken if air is introduced during mixing.

CETEARYL OLIVATE/SORBITAN OLIVATE With the increasing importance of organic certification many companies use a combination of cetearyl olivate and sorbitan olivate, which is allowed in EcoCert-certified skincare products. The combination is available in the US and UK as "Olivem 1000 ™". It is obtained by combining fatty acids from olive oil with sorbitol and cetearyl alcohol. Sorbitol occurs naturally in fruits and vegetables and has humectant properties similar to glycerin.

Thickeners

CETYL ALCOHOL This fatty alcohol, derived from palm or coconut oil, is used as a thickener in creams and lotions in combination with emulsifiers.

CETEARYL ALCOHOL A combination of cetyl alcohol and stearyl alcohol—two vegetable-derived fatty alcohols that act as emulsifier and thickener in creams and lotions. Cetearyl alcohol can often be used instead of cetyl alcohol, though it produces a heavier cream.

Detergents

GLUCOSIDES A group of surfactants produced from renewable raw materials (corn and coconut) that are mild and readily biodegradable. The group includes coco glucoside, decyl glucoside, and lauryl glucoside, sometimes sold individually or in pre-mixed blends.

COCOMIDAPROPYL BETAINE A mild surfactant derived from coconut oil. It is often used to make the product foam more and to improve the viscosity (thickness) in shampoo or shower gel formulations.

SODIUM COCOSULPHATE This contains purified fatty alcohols derived from natural coconut oil. It is a mild surfactant that gives a dense, rich lather and adds conditioning qualities and viscosity to shampoo and shower gels.

SODIUM COCOAMPHODIACETATE An extremely mild, highly foaming surfactant derived from coconut oil for a soft, conditioned after-feel to skin and hair; ideal for sensitive skin.

PLANTAPON SF A blend of (INCI) sodium cocoamphoacetate, glycerin, lauryl glucoside, disodium cocoyl glutamate, and sodium lauryl glucose carboxylate that complies with EcoCert standards for natural and organic cosmetics. A mild surfactant mixture it has good foaming properties and can be mixed with water to create shampoo, shower gels, and bath foams. It is used with Lamesoft (also called Natural Fat Restorer), a blend of coco glucoside and glyceryl oleate that is also EcoCert approved and acts as a combined thickener and moisture-restoring agent.

Preservatives

Many preservatives available to the home crafter come as pre-mixed blends, so I advise researching what is available in your home country.

PHENOXYETHANOL, ETHYLHEXLYGLYCERIN These are synthetic preservatives derived from grains and plants. Phenoxyethanol is considered one of the least irritating cosmetic preservatives and is effective over a wide spectrum of bacteria, as well as inhibiting yeast and mold. Ethylhexylglycerin reduces interfacial tension on the cellular walls of micro-organisms, to help destroy them more quickly. This blend is suitable for creams and lotions and is effective across a wide pH range. It cannot be used in detergent-based products.

BENZYL ALCOHOL, PHENOXYETHANOL, POTASSIUM SORBATE Benzyl alcohol is a common ingredient in fragrance due to its pleasant rose-like odor. Phenoxyethanol is explained above. Potassium sorbate is a common food preservative considered safe for use in natural and organically certified skincare products, but it can be a skin irritant.

LEUCIDAL A fairly new and seemingly more natural preservative available in the US; I have not managed to find a small-scale UK-based supplier so have not yet tried it.

PHENOXYETHANOL, CAPRYLYL GLYCOL Phenoxyethanol is explained above. Caprylyl glycol is a humectant with antimicrobial activity, so it has the additional benefit of providing a great skin feel to your products.

Resources

I run perfumery classes in the UK and have online classes for those who can't attend in person. Dates and venues can be found on my blog here:www.karengilbert.co.uk

OTHER WORKSHOPS:

www.trillfarm.co.uk Trill Farm is set in 300 acres of beautiful hills and woodland on the Devon/Dorset border. Owned by Romy Fraser, the founder of Neal's Yard Remedies, it provides the opportunity to learn sustainable living skills for the future including classes in health and wellbeing, sustainable living and craft, ecology and environment.

www.aromantic.co.uk Natural skincare product making classes in the UK.

formulabotanica.com Online courses in natural skincare product formulation.

FURTHER READING AND FORUMS:

swiftcraftymonkey.blogspot.com This is a fabulous blog full of good information on making your own products. I also recommend her downloadable e-books which are packed with information and simplify the science bits.

www.forum.fresholi.co.uk A very friendly UK-based forum for people making their own soap and cosmetic products.

www.thedishforum.com/forum A popular US soap and cosmetics making forum.

www.ctpa.org.uk UK-based cosmetic, toiletries, and perfumery association.

www.fda.gov USA food and drug administration.

www.ifraorg.org The international fragrance association.

Saponification calculator

You will find a useful saponification calculator for use in soap making on my website:
www.karengilbert.co.uk/index.php/links-and-resources

Books

This is a list of books that I have on my shelf and refer to time and again:

AROMATHERAPY

The Fragrant Pharmacy
by Valerie Ann Worwood
The Fragrant Mind
by Valerie Ann Worwood
The Encyclopedia of Essential Oils
by Julia Lawless
Aromatherapy and the Mind
by Julia Lawless

HERBS

Bartram's Encyclopedia of Herbal Medicine by Thomas Bartram

OTHER

The Aromantic Guide to unlocking the powerful health & rejuvenation benefits of vegetable oils
The Aromantic Guide to making your own natural skin, hair and bodycare products
both by Kolbjorn Borseth of
www.aromantic.co.uk

Ingredients suppliers

Most suppliers listed below sell a range of natural oils, fats, and waxes to make your own products. Do shop around as some sell ingredients that the others may not and prices do vary.

UK

www.fresholi.co.uk
Essential oils, butters, and waxes – great prices, quality and customer service.

www.aromantic.co.uk
Herbal ingredients, preservatives, natural surfactant base (Plantapon), natural fat restorer (Lamesoft), preservatives and emulsifiers.

www.thesoapkitchen.co.uk
Good value for basics such as bicarbonate of soda and citric acid as well as a range of emulsifiers, oils and butters.

www.naturallythinking.com
Aromatherapy supplies and my favorite for jars and bottles.

www.gracefruit.com
Oils, waxes, and butters plus great lip balm tins.

www.nealsyardremedies.com
Good-quality essential oils and herbs.

www.aqua-oleum.co.uk
Good-quality essential oils and aromatherapy supplies (owned by Julia Lawless).

www.baldwins.co.uk
Dried herbs and herbal tinctures.

USA

Being UK based I have not ordered from these companies myself, but all have been recommended on many of the US-based forums and sell an extensive range of oils, waxes, emulsifiers, preservatives, and surfactants.

www.teachsoap.com
www.brambleberry.com
www.makingcosmetics.com
www.theherbarie.com
www.lotioncrafter.com
www.wholesalesuppliesplus.com

Index